REACH YOUR COMMUNITY

Through Basketball and Other Sports Programs
A Guide to Energize and Unify Your Neighborhood Through Sports and Related Volunteerism

Written by Hosea James Givan II

Foreword by Nate "Tiny" Archibald

Afterword by Stu Jackson

Edited by Jean Marie Givan

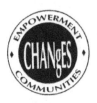

What people are saying about *Reach Your Community*!

"For the 40+ years that I've known him, Hosea has always been at the forefront of Youth and Community Empowerment. Long before Obama made it cool to be a community organizer, Hosea was in the trenches with rolled-up sleeves - year in and year out - doing the much needed work to pull us all up and through. His passion, drive and steadfast dedication to living and leading a life of service has been a shining example for me and for those lucky enough to have crossed his orbit!. If you've ever doubted that one person can make a difference, Reach Your Community is proof-positive that one person certainly can - and the culmination of a life well lived and grace defined."

- Gerry Erasme, Retired Sports Marketing Director for NIKE North America

"I have known Hosea Givan since our college days (Long Island University). As long as I've known him he has always been involved in youth basketball. The appreciation he has for our youth is tireless. Coaching, starting youth programs, and empowering young people to do better have always been his main focus throughout his career. Embarking on his new adventure, this book "Reach Your Community" is a solid guide for volunteerism in your local community. A must read for community volunteering!"

- Flora Krind, Retired New York City Police Officer

*"Hosea Givan says, '**Give back** can't be buzzwords or a hashtag.' This should really be his life mantra. Givan is doing the work that he was born to do and has ignited that spirit in those around him. With Reach Your Community, Givan is passing the baton to future runners by providing any and everyone with this manual on how to do just that - reach your community. He places the need in historical context and clearly outlines the how taking away any excuses for not being engaged, for not doing the work. This is not just required reading for volunteerism, it is required reading for the survival of our communities."*

-Maria DeLongoria, Ph.D., Chair, Department of Social & Behavioral Science, Medgar Evers College - CUNY

"Mr. Givan has been volunteering and serving our youth for over 40 years. This book provides the blueprint on how sports and basketball can be used as a guide to impact the future of our youth and community positively."

- Derek Phillips, Founder and Executive Director of Real Dads Network

"I have known and known of Hosea for a great many years from our days in New York. Throughout this time, he has always exhibited a passion for service of community, dedication and support for his fellow man/woman, as well as, displaying a great penchant for youth athletic engagement and participation. In addition to his book being an extension of his commitment to service, it should also serve as a protected historical document that is full of gifted anecdotal information to guide those seeking to make a difference within their community, regardless of whether it be of an athletic or non-athletic endeavor. Hosea, thanks for bringing to light such an awesome roadmap for community engagement, structure and success."

Jeff Hood, CEO
National Association of Police Athletic/Activities Leagues, Inc.
(National PAL)

"For years, sports have been a vehicle in urban communities that have created options for our youth to place within their reach opportunities that they never before dreamed possible. The work that Hosea has done for decades with countless young people has had a tremendous effect. I met Coach Givan in the 7th grade and played under his direction for 5 years. The lessons that he shared with me and have now finally placed in the pages of this book are life-changing and should be applied by any person working with our community's youth. Kudos to him for finally sharing the formula that has helped me and so many others. We will all be better for engaging this work using Hosea's model."

Charles F. Coleman, Jr.
Civil Rights Attorney, Legal Analyst for BBC, MSNBC, CNN and TYT

Hosea Givan is the epitome of a selfless and committed leader who perfectly demonstrates how sports, society, community and mentoring can powerfully intersect for the betterment of the people. From fatherhood to being a husband, from coaching to inspiring, Hosea shows us that hope with a plan for success can unite. "Reach Your Community" is not just a blueprint in how to take the steps to bring harmony to your neighborhood; it is the roadmap necessary to show our people how to create generational impact that empowers our communities for generations to come.

Michael Blake, Former New York State Assemblymember
Twitter: @mrmikeblake
IG: mikeblake1922

ISBN: 978-0-578-877723-5

"How blessed we are to take part in the positive development and progression of our youngsters."

- Carmen Morris-Givan

Dedications and Acknowledgements

I dedicate this book to my wife and partner, Rachel, and our daughter, Rebekah. I also dedicate this book to my mother, Carmen, who taught us early to love our community, help others, and my father, Hosea. He was and is an excellent example of a community servant. My life ambition was to make a difference in the world, as they did. As I have throughout my life, I will keep working hard to make them proud.

In addition, I dedicate this book to my first comrades in community service: my brothers, Gerald and Michael, and my sister, Jean Marie. Each of us has reached different communities in one way or another. We have been accountable for the values instilled in us as children.

I want to acknowledge Cecil Hollar, George Northcroft, Wes Yearwood, Nate "Tiny" Archibald, Ernie Rudloff, Al Vann, Gil Reynolds, Curtis "Mr. T." Thomas, Kimberly Adeduku Amerbor Reese (My publicist), Milton Carter. Jr., Ted Gustus, Jr., Scott Pierce, Joyce Myers, Rev. Jeffrey L. Smith, Nayron Monk, Cornell Fowler, James Coursey, Howie Evans, John Johnson, Sr., Dominic Jenkins, Charles Thomas, Oswald Stubbs III, Leslie Daniels, Peter Smith, Donald Francois, Dorothy Barnett, Craig Phillips, Sr., Eugene Devore, Fred McKay, Robert Horton, Larry Golden, The Homeboys Athletic Association, Tony Dinkins, Chester Mapp, Howie Lawrence, Craig "Kat" Keyes, Andre Anselme, Gerry Erasme, The Boston Crew (Claude Pritchard, Keith McDermott, Robert Lewis, Greg Lawson, Santonio "Pumpkin" Gooding and Anthony Taylor), Yvette Danielle Ashleigh, Geovanni Rivera, Brother Kevin Cawley, Chris Williams, Mickey Middleton, Tre Mc Millan, Donald Hazelton, Robert Greene, Thelvis Alston, Debbi McKune, Henry Comas, Adele Armstrong, Dr. Maurice Henderson, Darryl Burgess and the many others who responded to my requests for the support over the years. Thank you!

Table of Contents

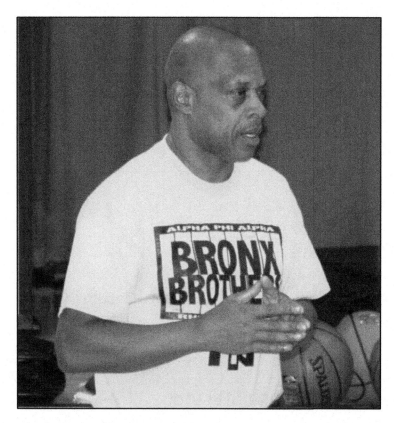

NBA Hall of Famer, Nate "Tiny" Archibald

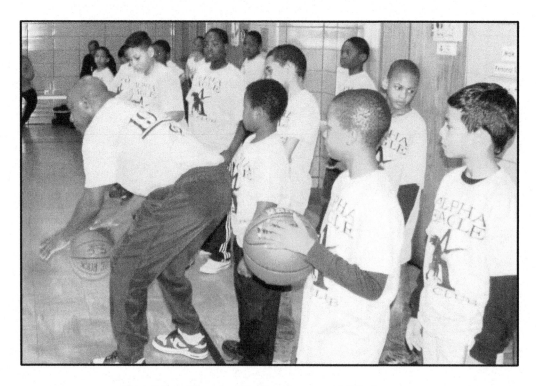

Teaching the youth the game of life!

Foreword

By Nate "Tiny" Archibald

Before playing basketball at DeWitt Clinton High School in the Bronx, NY; before playing college basketball at Arizona Western and the University of Texas-El Paso; before playing in Rucker Tournaments, before going pro and playing in the NBA, and before being inducted into the Naismith Memorial Basketball Hall of Fame, there was a local community where I was raised in the South Bronx (143rd Street and Morris Avenue). And that was just a piece of the puzzle or mosaic.

There was also a school, P.S. 18 (in the Bronx) and P.S. 120 (in Manhattan). Howie Evans, who wrote for the Amsterdam News, had tournaments. Cecil Watkins did the same in East Elmhurst. There were Floyd Lane, Hilton White, and many others. But it wasn't just the people associated with basketball. It was the community, plus the coaches, including police officers, firefighters, family members, and many others, who helped build a foundation.

When I think about Hosea and the programs he has been running, it reminds me of how it was when I was growing up and after I retired from the NBA. It caused me to reflect on some of the things I had been doing a long time ago in a very small community center. It wasn't even a legitimate gym. We were in the lunchroom, and we had makeshift baskets because we couldn't use the gym. I wanted to create the type of environment that was around when I was a kid.

I lived in the projects. Lots of bad things happened in and around the projects, but when you got to the community center, there were rules and regulations. You were in a safe environment. Your mentor (male or female) was advising you in ways that expanded your knowledge base beyond basketball. Basketball was the magnet that drew you to the community center, but you learned so much more once you got there.

People were conscious enough to say, "I'm going to spend time with these kids" because they didn't want us out in the streets and running around the projects, unsupervised, or being influenced by people who were up to no good – some of the riff-raff. There were good people in that environment but also lurking were dangerous temptations and perilous pitfalls. The community center was a place we could go and get steered in the right direction.

Nowadays, we're more aware of the ravages of the drugs that ran rampant in our communities than we were back then. We were naïve as to how drugs were destroying a significant part of the population, including many of our friends and relatives. People might think *you escaped the madness by going to Texas-El Paso. You played ball, you're good.* Well, we did not play basketball all of the time. Life lessons learned at the community center are some of the things that sustained me when I went to college and throughout other phases of my life. When we went to the community center, that was like going to school.

It was that type of environment at the school where Hosea ran his program. It reminded me of being a youngster again and learning the game all over again. It reminded me of when we had teams and leagues long ago. But we didn't have resources.

There was a time when I was coaching a team of kids from the projects. Nobody wanted these kids. They weren't that good. But I said, "I'mma take them" because back when I was younger, I don't think I was that good. That didn't stop me from getting better, though.

The skills and drills I was taught when I was a kid helped me to improve. I wanted to be better. I didn't want to be embarrassed. So, I could relate to those kids, and sometimes the hardest thing to learn when you get a little older is trying to teach other people what you learned.

But it's mandatory. Someone did it for me, and then it became my time to coach and mentor, even though our resources were sparse. We were out there for the kids, and the relationships that were built as I coached and mentored those children who are now adults remain to this day.

There were some other teams that those kids could not play on. They said, "We can't play for those teams, but we can play for you?" I said, "Of course." I didn't tell them nobody wanted them.

I was an introvert. So, I wanted them because of the experience. Not that I really wanted to get into coaching, but I wanted them and myself to have some identity.

People way back then were saying, "Man, you're coaching these guys?" I said, "Yes," because it gave me an outlet in the community. I was in school at the time, so when I came back around the block and went into the community center, it was expected. They would ask me, "Hey man, you gonna have a team this year? You gonna have a team this summer?" "Of course, I am, and I'mma pick y'all guys," I said.

One time, we had a game at the park on 129th Street, and because of the round robin, we ended up playing against Felipe Lopez, back when he was an All-American from Rice High School who played with the Gauchos. Of the guys 6'2", 6'3", he was "the man." He wound up in the NBA but back when he played against us. One time he dropped 50 points on us! My team ended up meeting up against him a week or so after that. Mind you, our team wasn't supposed to be good.

One of my guys let me know, "I'mma take care of this right now." Sure enough, he and the team did. I had seen Felipe not too long ago, and he remembered that and told me, "Y'all didn't have a good squad," but we held him. He said, "Your guys took me out." Felipe had dribbled the ball, went up, and that was the last time he played against us.

I let him know, "That was the pride message they were sending you that day. That you weren't going to get 50 on them again." It was a message that said, "Yes, we are from the projects, but we're not going to get embarrassed." That positive pride swell came from being a part of a community.

That's just one of many memories that come from having basketball and sports programs in our community. Use this book as a guide to help you create a safe environment for children, but not just a place for children. Bear in mind that it can serve the dual purpose of not only helping kids but adults can experience ongoing personal development in such an atmosphere, all the while enjoying fun, healthy athletic competition and forming lasting memories. Being a facilitator, coach, a mentor is exceptionally challenging but well worth it.

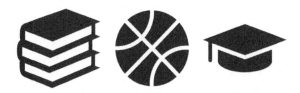

Nate "Tiny" Archibald

 6-TIME NBA ALL-STAR

 1973 LED NBA IN SCORING AND ASSISTS

 1981 NBA ALL STAR GAME MVP

 1981 CHAMPION WITH BOSTON CELTICS

 NBA HALL OF FAME

 WORLD SPORTS HUMANITARIAN
HALL OF FAME

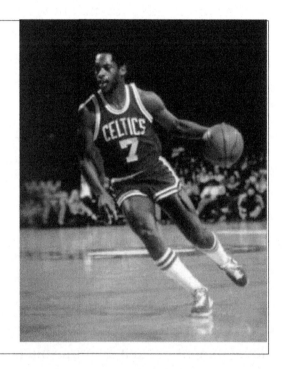

Preface

I let one of my mentees, Ozzie, know I was writing this book. I asked him to contribute. Here's what he had to say:

"When I first joined the Hollis Biddies back in 1994, I was one of the last players to come to the league due to the overflow of kids. It was about 11 of us if I remember correctly. Mr. Givan came over to us in the P.S 118 cafeteria and said, 'Hey guys, the teams were already chosen but I will make sure you have a coach and will get you all some uniforms.' He left us for about five minutes and came back with Coach Carter (RIP) and the NIKE P.L.A.Y shirts, for us. They both said to us, 'We take care of our own and will never leave anyone out.' That was the day I knew I wanted to follow in the footsteps of those positive black leaders.

Through the years, growing up with Hollis Biddies and not being the best ballplayer, Mr. Givan saw a different type of light in me and took me under his wing. To be honest, I can proudly say that without the life skills guidance and mentorship from Mr. G., I would not be where I am today. I remember a time when I was in high school, in the boys' locker room, a young Indian boy was jumped by a group of boys. When I came around the corner and saw the boy on the floor, I helped him up. Unfortunately, the boy thought I was one of the people who hurt him so the NYPD was called and I was brought to the precinct. When the school called my mother, my mother called Mr. Givan and he came right to the precinct to get me. He said to the officer, and I quote, 'There is no way that this young brother had anything to do with this situation, I've known him for a very long time and, hurting others is not in his nature.' That car ride back to my house with Mr. Givan was even more life-changing because he said to me, 'Oz, I know you didn't have anything to do with what happened because I know you. You are a leader and leaders will always help anyone in need.' That day, I will never forget. After high school and even to this day, Mr. Givan is still and will always be my mentor."

~Oswald R. Stubbs III, Operations Manager Hard Rock Café Atlanta

How do you reach your community through basketball leagues and sports programs?

One child at a time. Had I not established a rapport with Ozzie and his mom at the school where I went to kindergarten (P.S.118), in the neighborhood where I grew up (Hollis, Queens), via my community service through the basketball league I was facilitating, I would not have been able to boldly walk into that police precinct, defend Ozzie's character and insist he is released. The outcome could have easily gone another way. It happens every day. That's why you and people like you need to step up and serve in your community, making your presence known so when children need you, you'll be able to be there for them.

That was one of many instances that called me to intervene on behalf of children entrusted to my care. However, an incident on July 23, 2012, grabbed my attention and spurred me to do even more than I had already been doing.

I was in San Francisco for a conference. While surfing the 'net, I came across the gut-wrenching story about four-year-old Lloyd Morgan. A stray bullet senselessly killed Lloyd as a result of crossfire gun violence. Young Lloyd loved basketball. His parents affectionately called him "Little LeBron" and "President Obama." Sadly, he had his little life snuffed out before it began, another victim of the seemingly never-ending cycle of self-hate and self-destruction, running rampant through the streets of inner cities throughout America.

I felt like I was sucker-punched in the stomach when I realized that the horrific incident that forever changed Lloyd's family occurred three blocks from the school where I worked in the South Bronx. An eerie chill ran through my body when I turned and looked at my daughter, Bekah, who at the time was the same age as precious Lloyd Morgan, who had just lost his life.

My emotions vacillated, back and forth, between boiling rage and bottomless sorrow. Yet, I couldn't sit idly by and do nothing. After stewing for a few more moments, clear thoughts surfaced, and I sprung into immediate action. In no time, crafted an email and sent it to elected officials, and New York City Department of Education administrators. And any person with influence to whom I could connect, pleading with them to provide the necessary resources to renovate my school's dilapidated gym. In requesting those funds, I vowed to do everything within my power to help substantially impact that community, based on what I knew worked because of decades of such exposure, experience, immersion, and fruitful results. Through a basketball league with a life skills training component attached, I pledged to help usher in a needful change in that particular community.

A couple of weeks later, the then city councilwoman of that community, Helen Foster-McKay, responded to my email, committing $500,000 (FIVE HUNDRED THOUSAND DOLLARS, yes, half a million dollars) from the New York City Capital Budget toward the construction of an entirely new gymnasium!

"That's why you and people like you need to step up and serve in your community, making your presence known so when children need you, you'll be able to be there for them."

Where did I get the gall to make such an audacious request? What made me think I could fulfill that vow? Forty years earlier, as a young boy, I had a front-row seat watching a basketball league impact my Hollis community, the Hollis Biddy Basketball League (HBBL), also affectionately and popularly known as the Hollis Biddies. Men and women with a sense of urgency for the need to participate in our neighborhood's transformation came together. The ones involved were not unknown to me. It started with my dad, his good friend, and the beautiful people they assembled.

I knew what it took. I did not doubt that I could do it. I wasn't "new to it (using a basketball league to reach a community); I was true to it." Not only had I seen it played out under the leadership of my dad, the league's co-founder, and the dedicated community servants to the institution. I also replicated and enhanced the same model after I graduated from college and got my master's degree. It was in my blood, a part of my DNA.

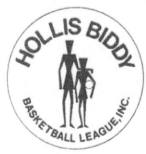

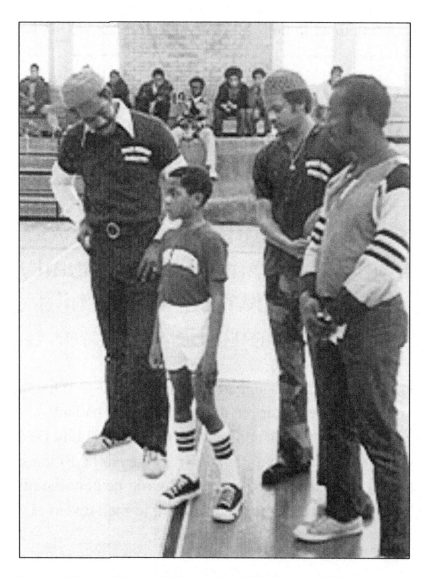

Hosea Givan, Bruce Bishop, Cecil Hollar and Don Averett

Introduction

My first volunteer experience came in 1973 when I was 13 years old. Based on the American Heritage definition of a volunteer, it means to be "a person who performs or offers to perform a service voluntarily." That being the definition, my first foray at community service was not technically voluntary, but I still count it as one.

Every Saturday morning, for three months in the spring, my father and many good-hearted, dedicated people ran a basketball league in our community, the Hollis Biddy Basketball League (H.B.B.L.). The adopted model for the Hollis Biddies was the East Harlem Biddy Basketball League, where my father and his good friend, Cecil Hollar, first coached, 1968 through 1970.

Recognizing the growing challenges in our own community, my father decided to bring things closer to home. The league was formed in our neighborhood in Southeast Queens in 1971 to provide for children an alternative to the drugs and gangs that infiltrated our communities, on the heels of the social unrest of the 1960s.

The league served children between the ages of nine through twelve. During that particular year, 1973, I had aged out of the league, and I was looking forward to catching up on some cartoons, old movies and sleeping in on Saturday mornings. However, my father was not going for that.

"You are not going to be lounging around the house watching cartoons while the rest of the family participates in the league," my father made clear to me.

My mom helped out with the girls' cheerleading program, which my sister Jeannie was a part of, and my two younger brothers, Gerald and Michael, played on teams in the league.

The position in the league that I was assigned to was as an assistant to George Northcroft. In his own right, Mr. Northcroft, a St. John's graduate, a member of Kappa Alpha Psi fraternity and a successful businessman, was an excellent role model for me. He assumed his role as head coach as if he were coaching the NBA's New York Knicks, with the utmost professionalism.

Mr. Northcroft gave me responsibilities with the team and made sure that I carried them out. In so doing, Mr. he gave me a sense of importance, and I felt like I was contributing to a more significant cause – and I was, even in the midst of my personal development.

I was in a leadership position as an assistant coach. I relished having that role, supporting the team and coach, and directing and encouraging the players under Mr. Northcroft's tutelage. I later found out that Dad saw to it that Mr. Northcroft directly influenced me, and it wasn't long before my brother Gerald was doing the same thing, under the watchful, caring eye of Mr. Northcroft, also.

Look at the circle of life. My dad entrusted his two oldest children to Mr. Northcroft. In like manner, Mr. and Mrs. Northcroft entrusted their two children, Dara and Martin, to one of Dad's children – Jeannie, who did some of her first babysitting, watching them on a few occasions. The level of trust and love in our families was high back then and remains intact to this day. As a result of the Hollis Biddy Basketball League, our families forged lifelong relationships.

Our team did well and made the playoffs that 1973 season. It turned out to be a fantastic experience, and when the season ended, I could hardly wait for the next one. And that initial volunteering opportunity was so rewarding; it set the stage for a lifetime commitment of "giving back." It's truly a part of who I am, and it's something I've been doing for over 40 years. And for the better part of my life, I have been encouraging others to make the world a better place through volunteering.

And what better time than now could this commitment to community service be more needful. We're amid a worldwide pandemic. A lot of activities have ceased. And a lot of people have gone inside, not just literally, but figuratively, as well. People are looking inside themselves and reconfiguring their lives.

While the COVID-19 has cost many people their lives, it's also given plenty of us who were not physically impacted by the Coronavirus a renewed sense of purpose and understanding that there is power in a focused, sustained effort for positive change. Once the pandemic is over, people will be free to release that stored up transformative energy.

One very troubling thing that is happening is prolonged isolation. The very nature of Covid-19 has people cut off from one another, which's vastly different from the world in which I grew up. I know it would be an excellent thing to re-create aspects of that type of existence once we reach herd immunity.

I grew up in a world where significant energy and emphasis were placed on community involvement, particularly as it pertains to children's basketball and sports lives.

My dad and Cecil Hollar, the Hollis Biddy Basketball League's founders, both worked at IBM. Those two incredibly charismatic men were able to attract the highest caliber volunteers. Men and women who held corporate executive positions, teachers, principals, police officers, health care workers, entrepreneurs, and even everyday, ordinary people of good quality. They were convinced and given by my father and Cecil the opportunity to "give back" by volunteering.

The level of support by the good people was outstanding. They came forward and stood up for our community by being there for the kids. That enabled young people and adults to have a safe place to gather to positively impact the lives of adults and children who still speak fondly of those experiences from decades past.

For the community of Hollis, the Hollis Biddy games first at Andrew Jackson High School, then Junior High School 192, was absolutely the place to be on Saturday mornings, from 9 a.m. until noon. There was a lot of "razzle, dazzle" as local kids played their hearts out, showing what they could do. And for those who were not as good as some of the others, they were evenly blended onto teams where they could experience some victories and simply play on a team.

Being a part of the league was not based on skill or talent. The budget allowed for 120 boys to participate. If a kid's registration was amongst the first 120, he was in!

Each kid was evaluated for their skill level and measured in height, so the league talent and height were evenly distributed among the twelve teams. A primary league rule was that each kid had to play at least one quarter, each game. Kids challenged one another because many of them had very impressive skills and performed at a very high level.

It was electrifying. The environment was warm, welcoming, and wholesome. It was such a wonderful mixture of children and nurturing adults who cared for them and neighbors who came to cheer on the league's participants.

Some notable Hollis Biddies Alumni include Darryl "DMC" McDaniels (of the hip-hop group Run-DMC), Jason "Jam Master Jay" Mizell (also of Run-DMC and was both a player and later a coach in the league), Jam Master Jay's childhood best friend Wendell "Hurricane" (a.k.a. "Cane") Fite who went on to DJ for the Beastie Boys and ex-NBA star, Lloyd "Sweet Pea" Daniels, among many others.

Former NBA star, head coach, and color commentator Mark Jackson played on the 1977 Hollis Biddies All-Star Team that defeated a Salvation Army team from Hempstead, NY (coached by the legendary Don Ryan, mentor of the iconic Julius "Dr. J." Erving). The tournament took place in Montreal, Canada.

A few years ago, the late Marie Jackson (Mark's mother) shared one of her special memories with me when we were back in the old neighborhood (at Jamaica Park in Hollis) for an MTV event. We were at a Hollis Biddies game featuring Rev. Run's son, Diggy Simmons. She recalled how Mark sank free throws at the end of regulation (with no time on the clock) to win the game for Hollis (and actually the U.S.A.) in the championship game.

Mrs. Jackson reminisced how she nervously was clutching my mother's hand during those highly suspenseful moments in the game. Mrs. Jackson spoke with such fondness and detail as if they played the game the day before. That experience with her is one I have come to cherish. A walk down memory lane is a good time to do other reflections.

A Bit of History

Derived from the African proverb "It takes a village to raise a child," the Biddies' slogan, "It takes a lot of people to raise a child," rang as accurately then as it does today. The societal climate that gave rise to the need of such organizations as the Hollis Biddies was the tumultuous 1960s. There were riots, much like there are in these days and times. That was in the era right after the assassinations of John F. Kennedy, Malcolm X, Robert F. Kennedy, and Martin Luther King, Jr. There was the Vietnam War back then. Now, we're still at war, maintaining a military presence in Afghanistan, Northwest Pakistan, Somalia, Northeastern Kenya, Syria, Yemeni, and Libya.

New Yorkers needed something to provide us a temporary escape from what was going on in the world at the time. Throughout the New York Metropolitan area, the 1970s was an exciting basketball period for our New York basketball teams. Who knew back then that we would classify those times as the Golden Years? The Knicks were *The Kings of New*

York," winning NBA championship titles in 1970 and 1973. Willis Reed and Walt "Clyde" Frazier were the stars of those Madison Square Garden based teams. The New York Nets, led by Julius "Dr. J" Erving, hoisted the ABA championship trophies in 1974 and 1976 at the Nassau Coliseum in Long Island. New York could boast about having champions in both professional basketball leagues! A winning basketball culture was ever-present in our town during that amazing era, and "The City Game" game gave us a much-needed distraction from the turbulent events of the 1970s.

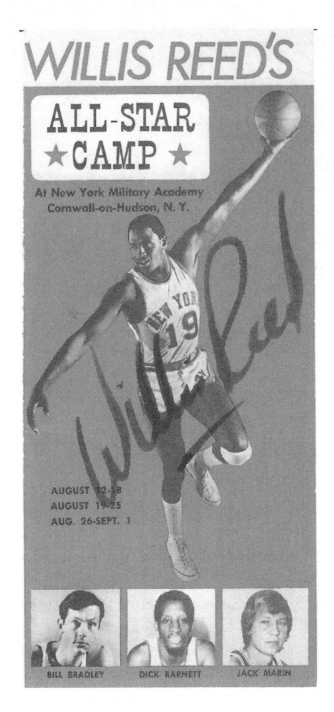

Each year the Hollis Biddies MVP received a free week at the Willis Reed Camp.

The Summer Rucker Tournament in Harlem attracted some of the best basketball players *in the world.* Playgrounds legends such as Joe "The Destroyer" Hammond, Earl "The Goat" Manigault, Pablo Robertson, Connie Hawkins, Herman "Helicopter" Knowlings, Richard "Pee Wee" Kirkland, and of course, Nate "The Skate" Archibald (as he was popularly known at the Rucker), generated frenzy level basketball entertainment "Uptown" in the summer!

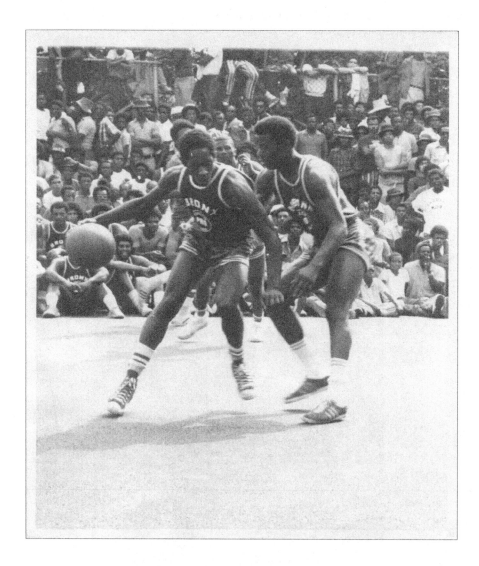

Nate "The Skate" with the ball at the Rucker Tournament in Harlem.

In local neighborhoods, basketball courts swelled to overflowing, standing room only capacity with "wannabe playground legends" engaged in fierce streetball competition! As you entered the park, you cried out, "I got next!" Then you waited until your turn and picked your crew to go to battle. And if your team lost, you might have had to wait for hours to get back on the court. Indeed, it was an extraordinary time, in New York City, for basketball. New York City was the basketball Mecca of the world!

Many young people back then had "hoop dreams" and were swept up in the exciting NYC atmosphere. We worked hard to make those dreams real, playing on the various neighborhood teams such as CYO, PAL, Elmcor, RVRO, Citywide, Night Center, I.S. 8, NYC Parks and Recreation, Brownsville Rec, Youth Games, and many others, too numerous to recall them all. The committed men and women who were willing to sacrifice their time, money, and energy to help give us something healthy and productive to do, allowed us to explore our dreams.

During those times, yes, there was massive sports program development. Still, national leaders (before their assassinations) Dr. Martin Luther King, Jr. and Malcolm X continually pushed for racial equality and fair treatment of Blacks while crying out against police brutality. Luminaries such as Angela Davis, Huey P. Newton, and Stokely Carmichael contributed significantly to bringing awareness of the needs lacking in our communities throughout the country, emphasizing self-determined community empowerment through voluntary involvement.

Though it is often pejoratively portrayed, the Black Panther Party originated in Oakland, California, created breakfast programs, community health centers, and taught the community to be self-sufficient. It was their strong stance against police brutality that contributed to their negative image in mainstream U.S. media.

Community leadership was strong, and volunteer participation in community activities was high! Community leaders were able to tap into the energy created through the movements of that era. The following attributes were dominant themes embraced by many American inner-city communities:

1. Helping
2. Giving
3. Building
4. Self-Pride
5. Community Pride
6. Sacrifice
7. Unifying for a Common Cause

It was necessary to pool resources due to scarcity.

Those times were the backdrop for the creation of the Hollis Biddy Basketball League. The electrified community energy coupled with the fact that basketball was at its peak of popularity in New York City made the task of motivating folks to help out with the H.B.B.L. so much easier.

For a while, such built-in motivators haven't been in place. In the 1970s, several movements (most notably: Peace, Black Power, and Women) naturally generated positive communal energy. The 1980s moved the world into being a "me" era, echoed in these days by the "selfie" generation.

The Civil Rights Movement that brought attention to the need for fairness and economic equality no doubt moved the needle. Consequently, many people made financial advancements and great strides. Despite that progress, something very unfortunate happened. Many people were consumed with upward mobility and took flight from voluntary community involvement and departed from those neighborhoods altogether, creating huge voids.

Whereas "back in the day," folks were willing to volunteer to coach or help out in other ways, organically. Before the pandemic, I noticed there had been a significant drop in the type of volunteerism that energized and sustained communities, as was the case when I was a youngster. People are so bent on "getting paid" that they do not schedule volunteerism into their activities. I absolutely am not against getting paid. However, at the grassroots level, genuine self-sacrifice needs to be felt.

Now, as we deal with this pandemic, so many things came to a screeching halt. Many people have had time to reflect. Due to circumstances beyond their control, people had to figure out how to reconstruct their lives. Many had lost loved ones, their jobs, and their sense of stability. We are encountering a historical stage of glaring food insecurity.

It's very harrowing, but I think we're at a pivotal crossroads during these historical times in which we live. It's time to press the reset button.

Technology has been a significant bridge used for people to connect, the Internet in particular. As we advance, there will be much more of the same. With the proper use of technology and other things to be mentioned in The C.O.A.C.H. (Challenging Our Adults to Choose Helping) Project™ Chapter, we can recapture and sustain a vibrant sense of community.

The primary purpose of this book is to SOUND THE ALARM, motivating and inspiring people to "give back" through volunteerism and creating and enhancing sports leagues throughout the world.

Tips for Getting Started Volunteering
First, ask yourself if there is something specific you want to do. For example, do I want...
* to make it better around where I live
* to meet people who are different from me
* to try something new
* to do something with my spare time
* to see a different way of life and new places
* to have a go at the type of work I might want to do as a full-time job
* to do more with my interests and hobbies
* to do something I'm good at

The best way to volunteer is to match your personality and interests. Having answers to these questions will help you narrow down your search.

Source: World Volunteer Web

Covid-19 has had people cooped up inside for more than a year. There has been severely limited interaction and outdoor activities. The shift in the community from physical to online and technological has caused some to survive the dreadful pandemic. Thankfully, there are medical advances that are helping to stem the tide. And one soon day, this will all be behind us.

Just as it was in the Hollis Biddy days, it is imperative for communities to band together, lock arms and provide environments that build children's character. Young people need positive role models that guide and nurture them. Leadership must demonstrate teamwork. When that happens, communities rise from the ashes, and we build a better society.

Adults who participate in such activities get an opportunity to engage in a purposeful existence while their own personal skills are enhanced—reinforcing good habits. Kids have a way of making sure adults are on top of their game.

As far as isolation in socialization goes, it can't happen in a thriving community. An old adage for one of the leagues we used to play in was: "Each one, teach one." Well, in these times, it's more about "each one, reach one." At least one, because nowadays (with the Internet) a reach to one could reach one hundred, one thousand, or one million.

Let me be clear, while it is important to have hopes for the best things in society and around the world as a whole, I have found it's best to break things down into bite-sized pieces to be able to develop and execute actionable plans. I have a particular focus that is near and dear to my heart: inner-city boys, who are often misunderstood, misidentified, misguided, and misinformed.

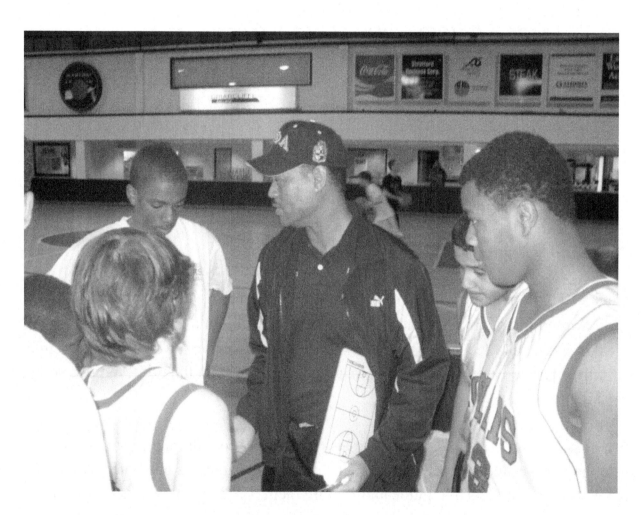

Coach Givan during a time out.

WE NEED MALE COACHES FOR OUR INNER-CITY BOYS!

They desperately need to be bombarded with more *positive male role models.* Our girls need this as well. I, however, utterly understand that it is vital for me to "stay in my lane." My calling and life emphasis have been predominantly to uplift our young urban male youth.

The ratio of players to a coach is usually about 12-to-1 for basketball. That is an excellent opportunity for one man to impact at least 12 lives. In greater detail, this perspective will be discussed later in the book, in The C.O.A.C.H Project chapter dedicated to the late John Wooden of UCLA and late Eddie Robinson of Grambling University, widely considered to be two of the greatest coaches of all time.

I've spent over 30 years as a New York City Department of Education public school teacher, guidance counselor, and dean. In that milieu, I gained treasure troves of experience dealing with inner-city youth. Additionally, I was an influential community leader and AAU basketball coach. Perhaps that's where I draw the "lion's share" of my knowledge in having my finger to the pulse as it pertains to today's youth.

With this book, I will give readers insight into what it takes to be a community leader and provide a better understanding of what it takes to impact the current generation through volunteer efforts, as it relates to basketball leagues and sports programs.

Although coaching basketball is the primary model used, most of this information could be applied to any sport, in any city, throughout America, and around the world.

If you have never coached or worked with young people, you can use this book as a tool to help you understand what is required for being a solid volunteer coach.
Stay tuned for upcoming webinars and other teachings I will engage in online and in-person.

The Hollis Biddies (which first ran from 1971 to 1982) resurrected in 1994 has been running strong in the community of Hollis, Queens, for the better part of 50 years. In fact, 2021 marks the 50th anniversary of the Hollis Biddies. Volunteer coaches continue to be the backbone of the organization.

In 1995, after witnessing what we created in Southeast Queens, my good friend and fraternity brother, Gerry Erasme, asked me to assist him in orchestrating a summer basketball league for the company he worked for (the international sneaker and sports apparel juggernaut, Nike). So, I went to work and produced a proposal for the Nike Swoosh Summer Basketball Tournament.

Gerry and I were the initial co-commissioners for what was then the largest summer basketball tournament in the country. During that inaugural summer, the tournament initially operated out of four NYC boroughs (Manhattan, the Bronx, Queens, and Brooklyn). Thousands of young male and female ballers benefitted from their participation in that resourceful summer basketball tournament.

With that same desire to reach and enhance the lives of children, I will utilize this book to provide information for you to use so you can reach YOUR community through basketball and other sports programs.

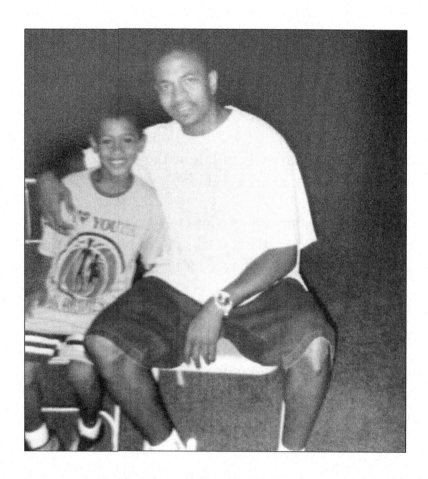

Mark Jackson and Hollis Biddy, Devon Pizarro.

NIKE SWOOSH
ALL METRO BASKETBALL TOURNAMENT

Biddy (Team Fee $150.)
12 and under, not thirteen (13) years of age before January 31, 1995.

Midget (Team Fee $175.)
14 and under, not fifteen (15) years of age before January 31, 1995.

Junior (Team Fee $200.)
16 and under, not seventeen (17) years of age before January 31, 1995.

Senior (Team Fee $225.)
18 and under, not nineteen (19) years of age before January 31, 1995.

Girls H.S. (Team Fee $150.)
18 and under, not nineteen (19) years of age before January 31, 1995.

* Tournament applications due Saturday, June 3, 1995.

* Tournament games will begin Friday, June 16th thru August 26th. (All teams will play approximately seven games before the playoffs.)

FOR MORE DETAILS CALL:

HOSEA JAMES GIVAN II. CO-COMMISSIONER

1-800-GIVE BACK

1995 NIKE SWOOSH ALL METRO BASKETBALL TOURNAMENT
108-53 62nd Drive (Suite 9A), Forest Hills, NY 11375

COMMUNITY SERVICE: Top 10 Reasons to Volunteer

Thinking of becoming a volunteer? See a list of reasons that will help you make up your mind.

#10: It's good for you.
Volunteering provides physical and mental rewards:
- It Reduces stress: Experts report that when you focus on someone other than yourself, it interrupts usual tension-producing patterns.
- Makes you healthier: Moods and emotions, like optimism, joy, and control over one's fate, strengthen the immune system.

#9: It saves resources.
Volunteering provides valuable community services so more money can be spent on local improvements. The estimated value of a volunteer's time is $15.39 per hour.

#8: Volunteers gain professional experience.
You can test out a career.

#7: It brings people together.
As a volunteer you assist in:
- Uniting people from diverse backgrounds to work toward a common goal.
- Building camaraderie and teamwork.

#6: It promotes personal growth and self-esteem.
Understanding community needs helps foster empathy and self-efficacy.

#5: Volunteering strengthens your community.
As a volunteer, you help:
- Support families (daycare and eldercare)
- Improve schools (tutoring, literacy)

Support youth (coaching, mentoring, tutoring and after-school programs)
Beautify the community (beach and park cleanups)

#4: You learn a lot.
Volunteers learn things like these:

- Self: Volunteers discover hidden talents that may change your view on your self-worth.
- Government: Through working with local non-profit agencies, volunteers learn about the functions and operation of our government.
- Community: Volunteers gain knowledge of local resources available to solve community needs.

#3: You get a chance to give back.
People like to support community resources that they use themselves or that benefit people they care about.

#2: Volunteering encourages civic responsibility.
Community service and volunteerism are an investment in our community and the people who live in it.

#1: You make a difference.
Every person counts!

(Center for Student Involvement, UC San Diego)

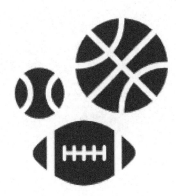

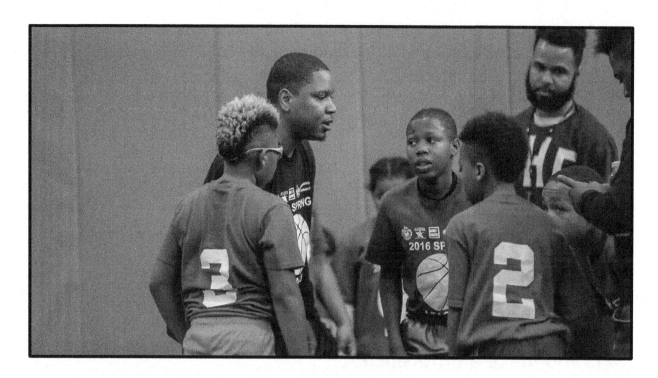

Coaches save lives!

WEBSITES FOR BASKETBALL COACHES

- Basketball for Coaches   www.basketballforcoaches.com
- Coach's Clipboard   www. coachesclipboard.net
- Pure Sweat Basketball   www.puresweatbasketball.com
- Teach Hoops   www.teachoops.com
- Coaching U   http://coachingulive.com

Chapter 1

Why You Should Start a Basketball or Sports Program

"Do you want to know the best thing you can do for a child? Give him or her some of your time. You might not be able to quantify this type of giving. There may never be a bottom-line calculation of the benefits. But the rewards will far outweigh anything your work can give you."

~John Starks, Former NBA Player

Ever since the Canadian American educator and athletic trainer, James Naismith, invented basketball (which was initially started with peach baskets) during the late 1800s to keep athletes in shape and relatively free from injury during the colder months between football and baseball seasons, basketball has become an excellent sport for athletes to develop physical fitness and many other skills. (1) Over time, basketball has grown into an international sport.

Harkening back to the impact the Hollis Biddy Basketball League had on an entire community, myself and many children in the area, I want to point out some reasons why YOU should start a basketball or sports program in your local area.

Kids Need Positive Role Models

I had the benefit of growing up in a two-parent household, and even with that, my parents had enough presence of mind to know how important it was to surround their children with positive role models. Children can become what they see. Especially when what they see is tangible, right before them, in real-time. They must encounter true success models to embrace and appreciate their reality fully.

With all that's going on in society, children genuinely need to see people navigating successfully through life. There are hostile forces (such as gang violence, bullying, drugs, obesity and increasing use of vape and alcohol, and many other vices) battling for the hearts and minds of our youth. What are YOU going to do? Sit idly by and not take action? Hopefully not! I believe you have a sense of the urgency and a heart to do some good on behalf of your community and children, or you wouldn't be reading this book. Again, I urge you to seriously consider putting together or supporting a basketball league or sports program in your area.

Children spend an excessive amount of time online, emulating social media influencers and music artists, some of who glamorize criminal behavior and "thug life." The absence of positive role models could have children copying who's in front of them. If it's you, perhaps you could put and keep a child on a positive path in life. That path might include being part of a team.

Basketball is a Team Sport

On a team, a child has a sense of belonging, being part of a unit. Young people, adolescents in particular, often need to feel that connectedness. It is one of the main reasons, so many youths gravitate to gangs. So many families end up fractured. Far too often, when a family structure breaks up, children are left flailing and ultimately severely neglected. That is a wide-open door for all types of vulnerabilities and perils. Children and community residents want to be a part of something beyond themselves, and sometimes something they don't find or feel in their own families. Creating a basketball league or sports program could help give them alternative and better options. A sports program is a solid choice. And the life skills of being a team player carry over into adulthood.

Playing Basketball Promotes Life Skills

When James Naismith created basketball, it started out having 13 rules. (2) Basketball (as it is now) still has plenty of rules. Those built-in parameters help kids learn that fundamental concept of "playing by the rules." That helps steer children into becoming law-abiding citizens who know how to respect authority. In these days and times, that could mean a matter of life and death for a child, especially for children of color.

There's absolutely no reason for some of the merciless and senseless killings of far too many youths whose lives may have been spared if they would have followed a simple directive given by an authority figure. Sometimes, it's an over-reach or abuse of authority or power, but if a kid is somewhat compliant, that might mean they make it home one more day. Crazy, but things learned in basketball and other sports-related situations can in some way play a part in a child remaining alive, literally.

"Giving back is essential to creating opportunities for the next generation. I've been able to be blessed by people giving to me, which allowed me to chase my dreams. It's only right that I continue to work to be able to give back to others."

—*Christian Vital (Memphis Grizzlies –G League Team)*

Kids Can Learn from Opponents

Besides learning from basketball how to get along and play with other teammates, basketball and other sports programs teach children how to face opponents and opposition. Life is filled with challenges and fraught with antagonisms and opponents; where better can a child learn how to deal with such life elements than in competitive sports? You can also help a child learn how to mitigate some of those challenges and draw parallels in real life.

Sometimes, the ups and downs of life translate into winning and losing, which are critical lessons of life that can be appropriately taught based on good coaching in basketball and other sports programs. It's not always about winning and being best that sometimes matters. It's also important to know how to face what comes against you. Playing basketball and being involved with sports programs helps develop that ability. And while skill, social, and emotional development are important reasons for a young person to participate in a basketball league or sports program in your neighborhood, why you should be involved is just as essential.

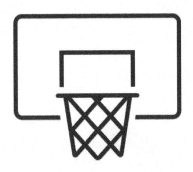

It's the Right Thing to Do

It's important to remember that if you have managed to make it to adulthood, more than likely, you have been helped by someone along the way. Whether you've been coached, mentored, tutored, picked up at home and taken to a game, sponsored to participate in an event or activity, or any other random, genuine, or intentional act of kindness, all those things count significantly! There probably is not a person alive who can say they have not been helped at some point in their life.

Discussing with my wife, Rachel, the notion that anyone who has been helped should help others, she connected the dots by stating, "that's everybody!" Which is so true. Everybody has been supported in one way or another by someone, so it's only fitting to keep it going by helping others. One of the best ways to help is by giving back.

Giving Back

Giving back is one of the most incredible things a person can do. "Give back" can't merely be buzzwords or a hashtag. It should be an immediate response to the needs that are so prevalent in today's world. Giving back unleashes the transformative power desperately needed in kids' lives that will impact those they encounter. Giving, like the Coronavirus, is infectious, and it could catch on – in a good way. When you give it back taps into that internal sense of obligation to return a good deed. That urge inside you to help as you were helped. It's there!

The collective force of that power can energize and enhance communities and negate destructive forces. It is not only based on love for one's community. It is also rooted in love for oneself. It's something the legendary R&B singer Marvin Gaye sang about in one of his songs, "Only love can conquer hate." He wrote those lyrics at a time when our country was erupting due to the social unrest bubbling over from the '60s and into the early '70s. It was true then, and it's true now. Maybe it could be you to start or run a basketball or sports program. I guarantee over time; there will be some "receipts" that prove what you have done has been worthwhile and worth your time.

"Coach Givan welcomed my family into his world. We were a white family from Williston Park on Long Island. My two sons played for him. Because of that experience, they are comfortable around, all people and it happened in a pretty natural way, through basketball. I will always appreciate one of the most valuable lessons in life. He taught my sons through his example that people are people and good people are good people."

–Donald Hazelton, Sr., Esq. (Professor, St. John's University)

Promotes Diversity and Inclusion

Sports activities allow young people to interact in an environment that can be used to celebrate and value diversity. Sports can encourage inclusion and the equal participation of underrepresented groups. (3)

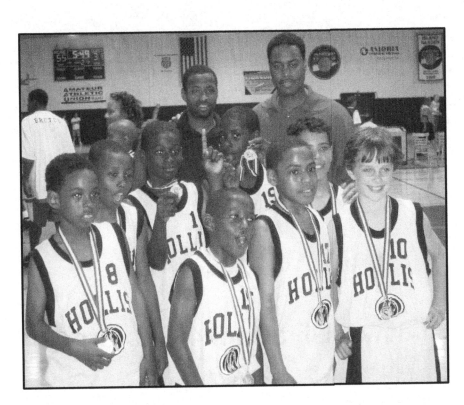

From left to right: Patrick Jackson, Christian Vital, Elijah McNeely-Davy, Khari Harvey, Rajien Griffin, Elijah Cokley, Thomas O'Connell and Donald Hazelton, Jr.

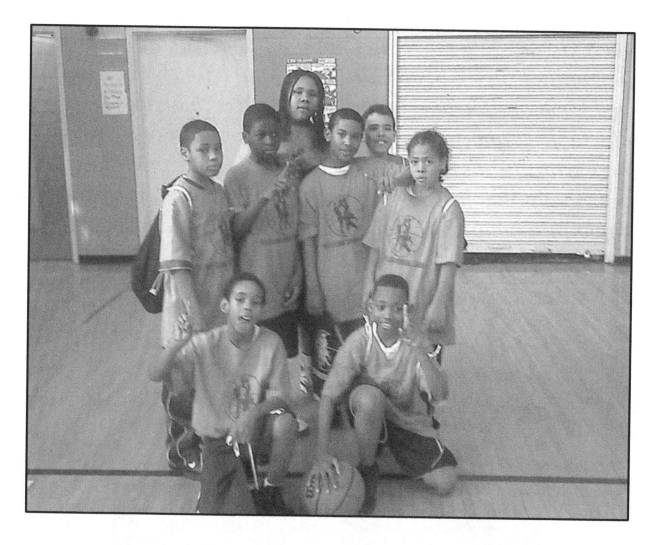

From left to right: Elijah Cokely, Patrick Jackson, Elijah McNeely-Davy, Cheyenne Gloster (the only girl), Devonte Green, Thomas O'Connell, Christian Vital and Naim Smith.

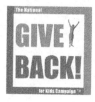

www.GiveBack4Kids.org

Chapter 2

Receipts

A few years ago, I got the text below from one of the young men I coached. I kept it as a memento, reminding me of the impact sports or youth activities can have on a child's development. It helps keep me motivated and knowing that I'm moving in the right direction when I stay involved with helping to uplift communities through basketball and sports programs.

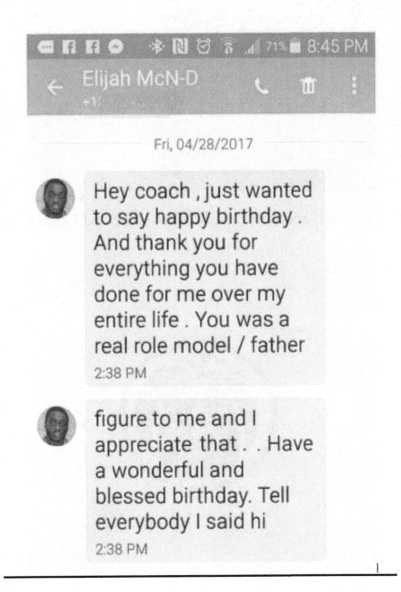

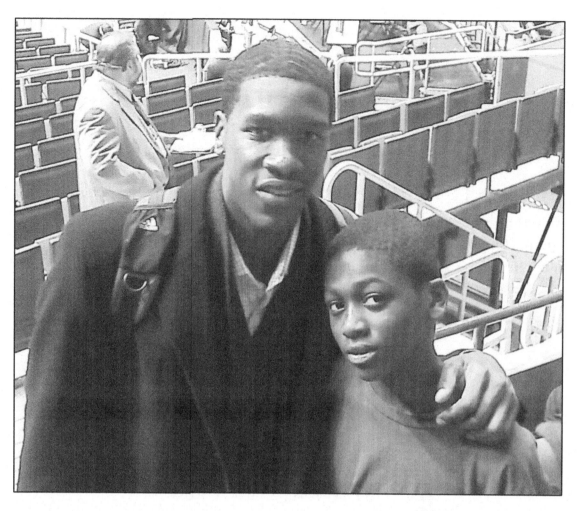

Brooklyn Nets Coach and Hollis native, Royal Ivey and Elijah McNeely Davy

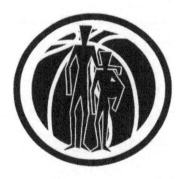

| Elijah McNeely Davy |

I was extremely excited to start the school year at P.S. 118 in the fall of 2004. I relished being in the role of dean at the school where, as a five-year-old, I began my formal educational journey and resurrected the HBBL. Our Hollis Biddies Saturday program was making its mark at the site. However, that's not what had me giddy! I was bubbling with anticipation at the idea of developing a highly competitive third-grade basketball team. In placing two particular third graders on the fifth-grade team, I had coached the previous summer, I made a wonderful discovery! I prophesied that the school's two "Elijahs" would be the foundation of an exceptional third-grade basketball team.

In assessing both boys' social and emotional needs, I knew that Elijah McNeely would require more broad support. So I decided to take him under my wing.

Elijah Cokely lived in a huge house a couple of blocks from the school with his mother, aunt (mother's sister), uncle, and cousins. It was a beautiful, immaculate home and a very stable environment with three gainfully employed adults. In stark contrast, Elijah McNeely lived with his mom, who wasn't working at the time, brother and sister, in an unkempt apartment located up the street from the Long Island Railroad Hollis train station. After visiting Elijah McNeely's home, comparatively speaking, it was an obviously far less stable environment than Cokely's.

School-wise, Elijah Cokely was strong, focused and confident, academically. Elijah McNeely, on the other hand, struggled and was more insecure regarding his academic ability. Both Elijahs were charming, good-looking kids who seemed wonderfully comfortable in their own skin. Their teachers loved them! Their mothers were raising both boys, and their dads were remotely in their lives.

In assessing both boys' social and emotional needs, I knew that Elijah McNeely would require more broad support. So I decided to take him under my wing, knowing that he would be a sort of special project within the project. My personal goal for all my players was to get them into college. I knew that if that were to happen for Elijah McNeely, it would require special attention on my part and others, "The Village."

Two or three times a week the first couple of years, I would meet Elijah in the school gym at 7:30 a.m. to work on basketball drills before school. I am not a morning person, so losing that extra 45 minutes of sleep was a huge sacrifice! The remarkable thing that stood out about Elijah's skill development was that he was ambidextrous. He was excellent at finishing a layup with either hand and was proficient at dribbling with both hands. Those are significant skill sets for any solid basketball player.

Elijah and I worked out a deal that I would work with his basketball skill development if he put more effort into his schoolwork. I would constantly try to figure out ways to help boost his self-esteem. I would really pump him up about his ball-handling skills and his ability to score with both hands. Most importantly, we talked about goals and the possibility of using basketball as a vehicle to get a college degree.

We would talk about college life, my fraternity Alpha Phi Alpha and the great men in the frat like Martin Luther King, Jr., Thurgood Marshall, Dick Gregory, Nate "Tiny" Archibald, and others. He met several of my fraternity brothers, including my good friend the aforementioned, NBA Hall of Famer, Sports Humanitarian Hall of Famer, and NYC basketball legend, Nate "Tiny" Archibald.

Elijah was excellent at finishing a layup with either hand and was proficient at dribbling with both hands. Those are significant skillsets for any solid basketball player.

I would say things to Elijah like, "I can imagine you living a nice house, married to a beautiful wife, and owning an impressive car someday. You are going to be an amazing father! All those things can happen to you. But you have to get this school thing down." Then I would ask him, "Can you see that for yourself?" And he would give me an affirmative nod with his million-dollar smile.

I would check in with him and his teachers a couple of times a day to gauge his progress. It was not long before I began to see an improvement in this attitude and a more significant effort in his academics. His confidence was starting to grow in that area.

Another positive thing that struck me about Elijah was his being an excellent big brother to this sister. I would watch him as he protected his sister, holding her hand while crossing streets as they came to school and returned home. That told me a lot about the kind of person he was.

By the late winter, we had assembled a strong third-grade team with Peter Smith's help, who became my main assistant coach. Peter was introduced to me by a mutual friend as someone who could help me develop a strong basketball program. Pete had a second-grade son, Naim, a pretty good player and one of the guards on the team.

My goal was to develop a strong third-grade team, good enough to qualify for the national AAU tournament in Orlando, Florida the summer of 2005. The tournament was held at Disney World's Wide World of Sports Stadium, the exact location as the historic and now famous 2020 "NBA Bubble." Preparing for that highly competitive tournament consisted of weekly practices and participation in local tournaments.

The team officially qualified to go to Orlando after successfully participating in the regional AAU tournament at the Island Garden run by Jim Foxx on Long Island. It was a significant first step onto the national scene for the Hollis Biddies basketball organization!

The Amateur Athletic Union (AAU) was founded in 1888 in New York City. It is the premier tournament in the country for young athletes in various sports (i.e., basketball, baseball, hockey, martial arts, track & field, volleyball, and wrestling). [4] However, out of all the sports, basketball is the one known in hoop circles worldwide.

As I was finalizing my rooster and expenses for the third-grade tournament, the team was hit with a bombshell. Unfortunately, Elijah McNeely was unable to make the trip because he had failed the New York State standardized English Language Arts (ELA) assessment and had to attend summer school. It was a devastating blow for our team. Elijah was one of our top players. However, eventually this, in part, turned out to be a blessing in disguise.

Our team went down and competed well, led by Elijah Cokely and Jaquan McKennon. We only won a couple of games and wound up in the middle of the pack, but we gained valuable experience for our basketball program. The coaches were pleased with the progress made that year and were looking forward to continuing building the program.

As it turned out, Elijah did not do well in summer school and had to repeat the third grade. We were able to turn that unpropitious situation to Elijah's and the team's advantage in the following school year. The AAU allows each team to have two "Grade Exemptions." A grade exemption allows a child who was repeating the grade to compete with their current grade. Many teams utilized the rule, and we were at a distinct disadvantage in Orlando because we did not have any grade exempt players on our roster. As I now see how Elijah's life has played out, this definitely was an incredibly positive turning point in his life.

Elijah Cokely's birthday was after September 1st, so according to AAU rules, he, too, was eligible to play on the third-grade team. The prospect of going back to the third-grade tournament in Orlando with our two main players from the previous year set the stage for an extraordinary destiny that awaited us!

For the third-grade basketball team, the 2005-06 school year followed the same pattern as the team the year before. We held practices twice a week, and the team competed in tournaments preparing for the AAU nationals in Orlando. That season tournaments extended beyond the New York City Metro area. We won several tournaments outside of New York City, most notably in Boston. Also, Elijah McNeely-Davy was then attending Huntington Learning Center on Long Island for additional tutoring. We were able to identify the necessary resources in order to make that happen. That was a significant move toward helping him fortify his academic skills.

We also added four excellent players to our rooster: Christian Vital (the son of one of my former Bayside High School players), Khari Harvey, Patrick Jackson, and Thomas O'Connell. After we beat Thomas's team in a New York AAU qualifying round, his dad approached me about Thomas playing on our team. After discussing it with my staff, we unanimously agreed to bring Thomas aboard. Thomas was a huge pickup. Naim Smith and Stephon Lloyd were the second-graders from the previous year that moved up. Amorri Waters was our lone second-grader.

On that Riverside Church championship team were three future NBA players: Donovan Mitchell (Utah Jazz), Eric Paschall (Golden State Warriors), and Ty Jerome (Oklahoma City Thunder).

We started to see the specialness of the team as we began to win more and more tournaments! The team's general manager, Harry Vital (Christian's uncle), produced a catchy Hollis Biddies rap song performed by a local artist, Gist "The Essence." Not many third graders had a song written about them. Those kids were neighborhood stars and played up to that billing!

The 2006 third--grade team we took down to Orlando to compete in the 164 team AAU tournament wound up *second in the nation*. We lost a close one in the championship game to the New York City-based Riverside Church Hawks. On that Riverside Church championship team were three future NBA players: Donovan Mitchell (Utah Jazz), Eric Paschall (Golden State Warriors), and Ty Jerome (Oklahoma City Thunder). Of our nine guys, eight played college sports, and all but one of those were in the sport of basketball. Christian Vital had the most successful college career. At UConn, he finished there among the top ten scorers in the school's history. Christian is now with the NBA's Memphis Grizzlies organization, playing for their G League team.

Our fourth-grade team was the top-seeded team in the AAU National Tournament in 2007. Our fifth-grade team qualified for the 2008 National AAU tournament in Memphis, TN, with a successful tournament championship at the Super Regional Tournament in Atlanta, Georgia. In the presence of his mother, who had since moved to North Carolina, Elijah McNeely played his best game ever as a Hollis Biddies baller, dropping 26 points in the championship victory.

Upon graduating from P.S. 118, I entrusted Elijah to my friend, Sandy Carter, a teacher and coach at I.S. 59. Elijah had a stellar basketball career and evolved into a solid student at I.S. 59. When it was time for high school, we chose Cardozo High School, at the time, rated as one of the top high schools in Queens. The high school coach there was another friend, Ron Naclerio.

I believed that once Elijah entered the tenth grade, I needed to have less of a direct presence. I felt it was vital for him to develop a greater sense of independence. He had to learn how to figure some things out on his own. It was finally time to create some space in order to for him to blossom.

I coached Elijah for the last time in the summer before entering the 10th grade (2010). We played in the LeBron James tournament in Chicago. Over the span of five years (2005 – 2010), our teams won 17 championships. Seven different players won MVP awards, which said a lot about the talent on the team. The boys worked extremely hard. Elijah won several MVPs, made many all-tournament teams, and became a nationally ranked player. In his junior year, he was the starting point guard for the New York City Public School Athletic League (PSAL) basketball championship Cardozo High School team. That was a huge deal!

In 2011, I tapped Elijah to play a starring role in the music video I scripted for the song "Give Back." I co-wrote the tune with talented, Atlanta-based singer Xavier Lewis. Although not commercially popular, most who have watched and listened agree that the song is a classic. In Philadelphia, the following year, the National Give Back for Kids Campaign conducted a spirited ten-city national tour with the music video promoting the spirit of volunteering, specifically to help our youth. That tour landed us on television in Philadelphia and Cincinnati. We were on the radio in Boston and Metro D.C. The music video is just one more thing that will eternally tie me to my former player.

Upon graduation from high school, Elijah attended and played basketball for Niagara County Community College. When he graduated from there with a B+ GPA, Elijah enrolled and played at Grandview University in Des Moines, Iowa. Des Moines is the same city where I attended college, Drake University.

While Elijah was in Des Moines, I utilized my network to help provide the support he needed. My fraternity brothers Broderick Daye and Phil Hall took him to dinner and went to his games. My dear friend Pop Wright, a former basketball star at Drake University, did the same. He also counseled Elijah and convinced him to "hang in there" at a challenging time for him at Grandview. I am proud to say that Elijah graduated with a degree in Sports Management from Grandview University, with a B+ average!

As I watched him play in high school and college, it was beautiful to see his growth as a person, knowing that seeds planted early on were sprouting into a well-developed young man. Along the way, I took some hits from coaches and players who believed that I favored Elijah. The truth is: it started with two Elijahs; both boys were warriors who I cherished, almost as if they were my own children. However, early on (by a type of paternal instinct), I realized the necessity of providing extra support for one Elijah due to apparent deficiencies. It was not a "Sophie's Choice" movie-type decision, wherein choosing one child, the other was destined for disaster. As expected, Elijah Cokely has grown into the responsible, self-sufficient young man I always knew he would become.

"As I watched him play in high school and college, it was beautiful to see his growth as a person, knowing that seeds planted early on were sprouting into a well-developed young man."

A few months after graduation, while living in Utah, Elijah McNeely signed a contract to play professional basketball in the Middle East. He arranged with the sponsors for me to go with him, as his father, to help him get set up out there. Upon further counsel, we decided against the Middle East professional league. We felt that it was best for him to stay stateside and pursue other overseas basketball opportunities. Until then, he will work on developing the entertainment company he created with his cousins, explore graduate school opportunities and if the opportunity presents itself, try his hand at becoming a member of the Alpha Phi Alpha fraternity.

To date, our ("The Village's") investment in Elijah has proven to be a fruitful one. His college graduation was a crowning achievement. He is well-respected by his peers and is known as a legendary ball-handler in parks across New York City. Through the years, we have remained close. I still look forward to seeing Elijah one day as a husband, a father, and a homeowner, driving a beautiful car. Something we both envisioned for him when he was just a third-grader at the gymnasium of P.S. 118 in Hollis, Queens.

Elijah, in his own words:
"Appreciate everything you have done for me over the years, coach. Love you like a father. And thank you for always being in my corner and guiding me down the right path."

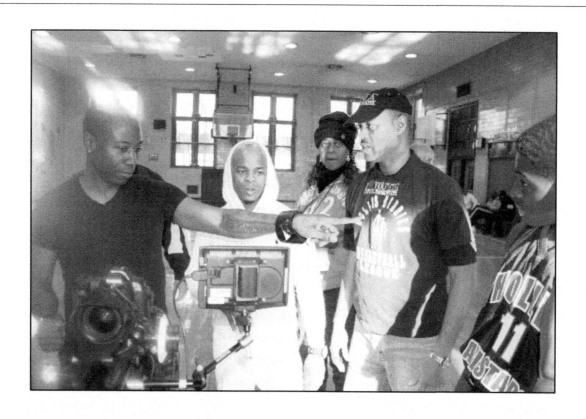

Elijah and Xavier Lewis star in the "Give Back" music video!
Check it out! https://youtu.be/1X2Dy-uOu2Q

There may be setbacks, but your efforts were not in vain!

| Charles Laws |

During the 2020 holiday season, I was in one of my nostalgic moods, as I often am these days. I posted on Facebook a picture of our 2005 third-grade Hollis Biddies A.A.U. team that went to Orlando, Florida. That was the inaugural A.A.U. team I mentioned earlier. I failed to note that it was modeled after a successful "travel team" called "the Homeboys" based in Forest Hills and St. Albans, which I coached in the mid to late '90s. However, my first bona fide A.A.U. club was that 2005 team.

The 2005 team picture surprisingly generated numerous positive responses from players I had not heard from in years. Among those players was Charles Laws.

I came to know Charles when I was dean at P.S. 118. Although he may have appeared cherubic, Charles was definitely one of the young men who gave me challenges due to his disruptive behavior. I was in charge of discipline for our school and certainly had to deal with Charles regularly.

Charles was raised by his grandmother and lived by the Long Island Railroad Hollis Station, a couple of blocks from where Elijah McNeely resided. Charles played in the Saturday Hollis Biddies program at the school and demonstrated better than average basketball talent. When forming the third-grade A.A.U. travel team, I thought that Charles would be a perfect candidate to play on the team. He eventually made the team which gave me some pretty powerful leverage with him school-wise to assist in his behavior modification.

The deal was for him to maintain his eligibility in order to compete in the national AAU tournament at Disney World. Charles had to be well-behaved and demonstrate strong effort in his schoolwork consistently. With Coach Peter Smith, Coach Donald Francois (my fraternity brother and other assistant), and myself, Charles was constantly in the company of positive men that genuinely cared about him. He truly benefitted from those relationships. In a relatively short period of time, upon Charles making the team, the school community began to see significant improvement in his attitude and performance in school. A win-win situation had been established between our school and Charles Laws. Everyone was happy!

The team went down to Orlando and did decently for the first time out. Charles scored some baskets in a couple of games, much to the delight of his teammates and the coaching staff. Charles had a warm personality, and the team loved him! We always took pleasure in his every success on and off the court. Charles was part of the crew that helped lay the foundation for the next third-grade team that would become both historic and legendary.

The following year as a fourth-grader, Charles and few others moved up and played on our newly created fifth-grade team, coached by Donald Francois. Coach Pete and I remained with the third-grade team.

Charles graduated from P.S. 118 and went on to I.S. 238, my alma mater. By eighth grade, we lost contact with Charles. No longer under our influence, Charles drifted back into unruly and unscholarly behavior. He attended Boys and Girls High School in Bedford Stuyvesant, Brooklyn, and later returned back to Queens at August Martin High School. Charles shared with me in a recent phone conversation that after getting "in trouble," he wound up in a juvenile facility for wayward youth, the St. John's Non-Secure Detention Center, in Queens. Charles never graduated from high school.

Unfortunately, Charles never developed the skills to play high school basketball and other skills he would have developed if he had a viable growth pathway. He was the type of kid that would have genuinely benefited from playing on community center or P.A.L. teams, like the ones that existed when I was in middle school and high school. Sadly, they did not exist at that critical middle school toward high school age for Charles. And those types of programs are still just as rare in the world today. Now is the perfect time to emphasize one of the themes of this book, "Young people can't play on a team if they don't have a coach" ~my own quote. Think about that and how Charles' life could have been less turbulent if there were more positive options available to him.

In a recent conversation, Charles shared with me that he still lives with his grandmother, now in Yonkers, New York. He is now 25 years old and does construction work when available. Charles has a girlfriend that he cares about a great deal. His favorite team is the Brooklyn Nets, and his favorite player is Kevin Durant. We had such a great time reminiscing about the "good ole days" and his helping me catch up with the lives of some of my former players. He wants to get his G.E.D finally. As the conversation ended, we promised to keep in touch, and I assured him that I would help him in any way possible to achieve his goals, short of me lending him money because I am on a retired educator's income these days. He laughed.

Charles really sounded stable. It pleased my heart to hear him express his appreciation for the time and energy we poured into him. I truly feel good about his future and, once again, recognize seeds sown produced an excellent harvest. Our words, actions, and concern for this player bore fruit. He is still growing, and our work isn't over.

Charles, in his own words:
"I never got to thank you for the opportunities you gave me and for not quitting on me when everyone else did. I will forever be grateful and forever love you for that."

It is truly a blessing knowing that I made a positive difference in someone's life. It's an absolutely beautiful feeling.

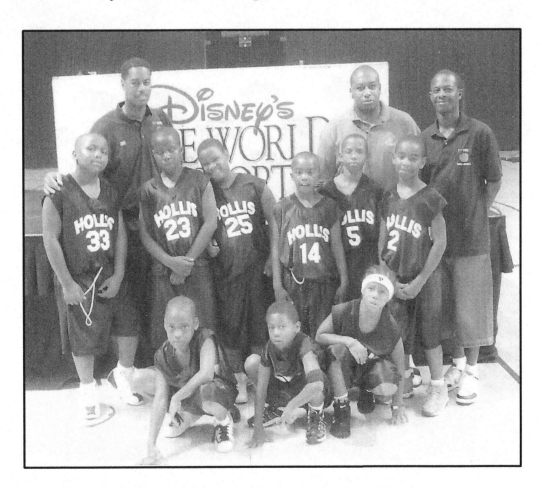

2005 Orlando Team (Charles Laws 3rd from left)

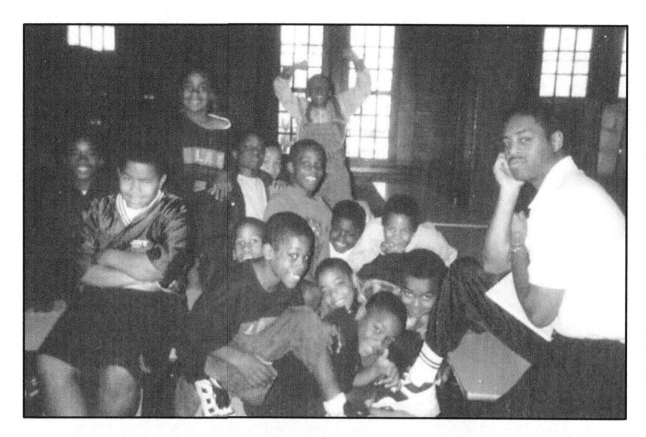

Ozzie as a Child (closest to my knee)

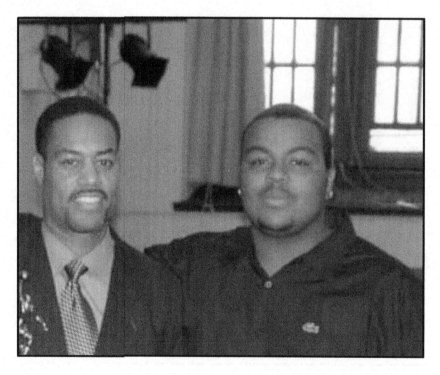

Ozzie as a Young Man (19 years old)

Sow the seeds and watch them blossom!

| Coach Ozzie |

Unlike Elijah and Charles, I never personally coached Oswald R. Stubbs III. Ozzie, as he is affectionately known, and his sister Donneqwa participated in the Hollis Biddies Saturday Program in the mid to late '90s. Ozzie, whose words grace the preface of this book, played basketball, and his sister displayed her talents in our dance program. I made that distinction because we eventually had boys dancing and girls playing basketball in our Saturday program.

We had about one hundred boys in the basketball league in those early years of the second coming of the Hollis Biddies. Unfortunately, as the league's commissioner, I did not get to know every player in the league personally. However, I certainly made every effort to know most of them. Ozzie did not appear on my radar until maybe his second year. He was such a personable little guy and full of energy, as was the case for most seven and eight-year-olds.

Throughout his time as a player in the league, Ozzie never emerged as one of the top players. He was a decent player but always played hard. Ozzie always put forth a top-notch effort and demonstrated incredible "heart," an intangible "gusto" that is admirable and unique.

Leadership development is a focal aspect of my basketball programs. The best leaders can inspire courageous acts and help transform communities. You can teach leadership. Two critical keys are that the person must be open to receive training and assume a leadership role. Then others seem to have God-given leadership talents. I believe that Ozzie fits into a special category. We groomed him to take leadership roles within the organization, but I also think he clearly was blessed with natural abilities. So in his case, I would say he has a healthy balance of both leadership that was taught and leadership that was innate.

By the time he aged out of the league at 13, he was "chomping at the bits" to become an assistant coach. Ozzie was one of those kids that made you realize how much kids watch every move you make. This reinforces the fact that if you assume a leadership position involving young people, you should accept the understanding that you absolutely are a role model and should always act accordingly. Sometimes children are aching for that role model to emulate, and you may not realize that you are the one he or she may be studying at the time. Nor may you understand the positive impact you are having on a young person.

By age 15, Ozzie was a responsible head coach in the league with maturity beyond his years. At 17, he graduated from Flushing High School. Ozzie became a student at the Metropolitan College of New York shortly after his 18th birthday. When he was 19 years of age, he literally had the keys to the P.S. 118 building. I was no longer working there at that time and had moved on to P.S. 463. However, in the ten years, I worked there, I never possessed those keys!

Ozzie arranged a lunch meeting with the president of his college and the National Give Back for Kids Campaign to discuss the two organizations collaborating on projects in the Bronx when he was 20 years of age. And that once little guy was now 6-3 and 250 pounds!

Ozzie was highly ambitious and always eager to take on more significant roles within the organization's Saturday program in Hollis. Ozzie was an intrepid leader whose charismatic and reliable leadership style reminded me of the league's co-founder during the first era of the Hollis Biddies, the legendary Cecil Hollar.

After years of dedication and hard work, it was finally time for Ozzie to be promoted from the role of coach to a higher position within the organization. I could not wait to proudly promulgate that the 20-year-old Oswald R. Stubbs III was the deputy commissioner of the Hollis Biddies Basketball League. By that time, I had handed over the leadership responsibilities of the league to Coach Charles Thomas. His father, the beloved Curtis "Mr. T" Thomas, was part of that initial leadership team that ran the Hollis Biddies at Andrew Jackson High School in 1971. I groomed Charles to take the mantle and equipped him with the extensive operations manual that I had developed. Most of which is in the appendix of this book. Ozzie was to assist Charles.

Ozzie was a full-time college student, worked full-time at a TGIF restaurant, and he had a part-time job working his grandmother's hot dog truck outside of Yankee Stadium. His plethora of responsibilities prevented him from producing the quality of leadership needed for the league and to his own satisfaction. He realized his duties at the Hollis Biddies were lacking, and much to his chagrin, Ozzie resigned his position with the league.

Professionally Ozzie continued to blossom and take on more significant management roles within the restaurant industry. Ozzie is currently living in Atlanta and is the operations manager at Hard Rock Café Atlanta. We continue to take pride in Ozzie's growth and development. His potential remains unlimited, and we look forward to his future accomplishments.

The reflections on the lives of three young men who have come through our basketball program are just a sample of the multitudes of the lives significantly impacted by basketball and sports programs. I shared those stories so you can realize how vitally important it is for such programs to be available for our young people. However, they can only exist if people are willing to share their time.

STRICT POLICY NOTE:

I think this is as appropriate a time as any to discuss our policy on preventing child abuse. Almost daily, we discover more and more victims of child abuse that go back decades. Innocent young people who trusted the adults to protect them while in their care became the victims. An hour doesn't go by where you don't see a TV ad by a law firm requesting victims to come forward to be a part of class action suits against their abusers. A sad reality is that youth programs attract pedophiles. All volunteers must be screened.

I have always maintained a very hardline policy for adults supervising children. An adult is never allowed to be alone with any child at any time in any part of the building or outside the building. If ever discovered an adult violated this policy, that adult will immediately be removed from the program, and an investigation would ensue. There is zero tolerance in this area. No excuses. The policy is also made known to the youth participants and their parents. To date, extreme caution has prevented child abuse within my programs. I'm always on alert. I trust no one in this regard. Unfortunately, child abuse has been widespread in this world and stretches back millenniums. You can never be too careful!

Background checks can be essential. However, they only report those who have been caught. Undiscovered pedophiles are roaming free. When developing a youth program, take every precaution to protect our children!

HIGHLY RECOMMENDED!
Sexual Harassment Prevention Training Part 1 and Part 2

- https://youtu.be/sL7LwBsV9bM
- https://youtu.be/1za7gs9S2H0

APPS TO HELP KEEP YOUR TEAM OR LEAGUE ORGANIZED

teamSNAP	www.teamsnap.com
SPORTS SIGNUP PLAY	https://sportssignup.com
TEAMWORKS	www.teamworks.com
JERSEY WATCH	www.jerseywatch.com

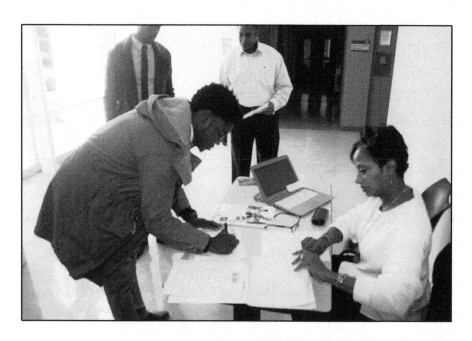

Registration

Chapter 3

Getting Started

"Start where you are. Use what you have. Do what you can."
~Arthur Ashe

The magnitude and depth of the challenges our communities are experiencing can appear overwhelming, to the extent, things may seem hopeless. Now is the time for imagination, imagining the impact of a successful program. Start with focusing your thoughts on succeeding in your endeavors. See the victory! Then put an actionable plan in place to obtain the desired outcome.

The first step is putting your plan together with pen and paper, or on your computer or whichever device you use, phone, iPad, whatever. Make it plain and attainable. I don't believe in limiting the scope of one's vision. However, there is nothing wrong with starting small and building incrementally over time. Sometimes starting small allows you to work out the kinks and establish a certain level of confidence and momentum needed to achieve the goal.

The next step is fortifying your knowledge for the task at hand. Take the time to understand all the intricate details involved in implementing the vision. Use learning guides, such as this one. Explore the internet for information. There is plenty of data available on this topic. Try to become an expert by soaking up as much intelligence as you can absorb. Please realize that "trial and error" or experience are the best teachers, however, use every source to gain information that specifically relates to what you're planning to do so you can be best prepared.

Building a Winning Team

To me, this is the hardest part of the journey toward creating a successful sports league. Identifying loyal and trustworthy supporters are the crucial ingredients in the recipe for a "delicious" sports program. Without this piece in place, you will never taste that sweet success you desire.

So how do you recruit your team? An excellent place to start is a school community where you may want to attract participants.

Many urban schools are without any sports program or any extracurricular activity. Most school leaders understand the value of such programs. Through sports, you learn teamwork, the importance of practice, discipline, how to win, and how to lose. Social skills are developed through direct and in-person interaction with teammates. These skills are essential when so many young people spend most of their social interaction in virtual environments.

"A good coach will help his or her team understand the correlation between getting along socially and winning on the court and in life."

A good coach will help his or her team understand the correlation between getting along socially and winning on the court and in life. Effectively sharing these advantages with the school team leadership should open doors towards forming a partnership. In most cases, you will need some type of reference. Find someone solid who can vouch for your character. Also, you should provide some form of a background check on yourself. As I mentioned in the last chapter, properly screening all volunteers is essential. It helps to protect our youth and the integrity of your vision. Thus, it would be best if you led by example.

Once you passed the first test by being accepted by the school leadership, you now have access to what could be your initial pool of volunteers, the parents. The parents of the participants could be your primary source of support. This also creates a great opportunity in terms of helping to develop community leaders. Often, adults are looking for ways to help their community but may find it challenging to connect with the right opportunity. Many parents benefitted from being involved with a sports program. Presenting them with the chance to "give back" may activate a seed planted in them when they were younger.

Local churches are another excellent source. Finally, as it relates to recruiting volunteers, don't ignore your own personal network of family and friends. They are probably inclined to share your values and beliefs and may be willing to help support your vision.

Partnering with a school could potentially solve the question of a sports facility. Using the gym or field could be a possibility. However, there could be costs involved, and those costs should be factored in when creating a budget. Here's an example of line items in a potential budget:

1. Uniforms
2. Space Rental
3. Insurance
4. Trophies/Awards
5. Equipment (i.e., balls, whistles, scorebooks)
6. Officials/Referees/Umpires

I have seen programs, including my own, attempt to reduce expenses by eliminating the final budget item "Officials/Referees/Umpires" and instead use parent volunteers in those roles. Officials, referees, and umpires are specially trained to maintain structure during the course of a game. In doing so, it also helps towards maintaining civility amongst the spectators, usually the parents.

If tight order isn't maintained in a game situation, the results could be disastrous. If you are planting your program in an urban setting, there is a good chance many people of that community live daily in a highly stressful environment. Unfortunately, many don't have or are limited in exploring ways to channel that stress in a more positive manner. Therefore, a regular youth sporting event could be highly combustive due to tensions created by societal factors. If at all possible, raise the money to allow for the best officiating of the game. Many headaches could be saved with the right people overseeing the flow of the games. Trust me on this. I learned the hard way!

Fundraising

Fundraising is another critical aspect of building an effective sports program. One straightforward way to raise money for your program is to offset the cost by charging the participants a program fee. You simply add up the costs and divide it by the number of players in the league. Unfortunately, doing so could eliminate the overwhelming majority of the young people that need it the most. Developing a fundraising plan could remedy that problem.

One suggestion would be to identify businesses within the community to help sponsor the program. Those local businesses and the entire "village" will benefit by having the young people engaged in positive activities. Please encourage them to invest in our future, the safety and well-being of local areas. I also want to emphasize the importance of tight fiscal accountability. Please delegate someone extremely trustworthy to manage the resources raised. The wrong person in charge of the money could cause your vision to come to a screeching halt.

Fundraising should be an ongoing process. Google various ways to raise money for the sports program. There are plenty of good ways to do so. And once you're ready to get things rolling, make sure you get off to a good start; you only have one chance to make a first impression. And once you begin each season, make it memorable.

Engage Your Community at the Year's Outset

Each year, in Hollis, we kicked off our season with a fun and electrifying parade celebrating the program's start. Our goal with the parade was to infuse positive energy into the community and our program participants. Our parade started at the corner of Hollis Ave. and Francis Lewis Blvd., our Hollis community's epicenter. In securing the necessary parade permit, New York City police officers protected us from moving vehicles and guided our 150-person procession down Hollis Ave. to 109th Ave., onto our final destination, P.S.118.

Marching down the westbound side of Hollis Ave., I vividly recall hundreds of appreciative Hollis residents (young and old) gathered along the parade route proudly cheering us on! We attracted the crowds because of the energized chants and music that could be heard from several blocks away.

I was always at the head of the parade and assumed the critical role of leading the chants. Before we started the parade, we always rehearsed the typed-out chants, so everyone was in sync. We never had the traditional marching band, so our children and volunteers were our parade stars. Each year when I donned the mic walking backward alongside the vehicle with the booming speaker system, I knew our parade started only three blocks away from where the legendary Run (Joey Simmons of Run-DMC) once lived. That realization always got me extra pumped! With a mic in my hand and with all the energy and enthusiasm I could muster, as the legendary Rakim once commanded in his famous rap lyric - I "MOVED THE CROWD!!!"

Me: Who's kids are the best!?!
Crowd: HOLLIS B-I-D-D-I-E-S!!!
Me: Who's kids are the best!?!
Crowd: HOLLIS B-I-D-D-I-E-S!!!
Me: When I say Hollis!
You say Biddies! Hollis!
Crowd: Biddies!
Me: Hollis!
Crowd: Biddies!
Me: Hollis!
Crowd: Biddies!
Me: Who's house! (From the famous rap Run lyrically boasted!)
Crowd: Our house!
Me: Who's house?
Crowd: Our house!

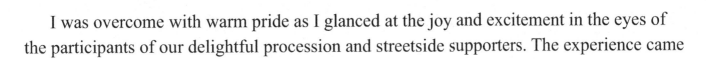

I was overcome with warm pride as I glanced at the joy and excitement in the eyes of the participants of our delightful procession and streetside supporters. The experience came to a beautiful crescendo when we arrived at our final destination, the program's site, P.S. 118!

P.S. 118 was up the block from "The Rock" at the intersection of Farmers Blvd. and Liberty Ave. The famous red, black and green (Colors of the Black Liberation flag) painted rock is a prideful landmark in the community where I grew up. Neighborhood icon, LL Cool J, featured "The Rock" in one of his music videos. Legend has it that Tupac Shakur's (hip hop icon) mother, Afeni, was instrumental in getting the rock painted in the 1970s when she was a member of the Black Panther Party. This story was once told to me on the J Train by the late activist Sonny Carson, on our way to Brooklyn from Queens.

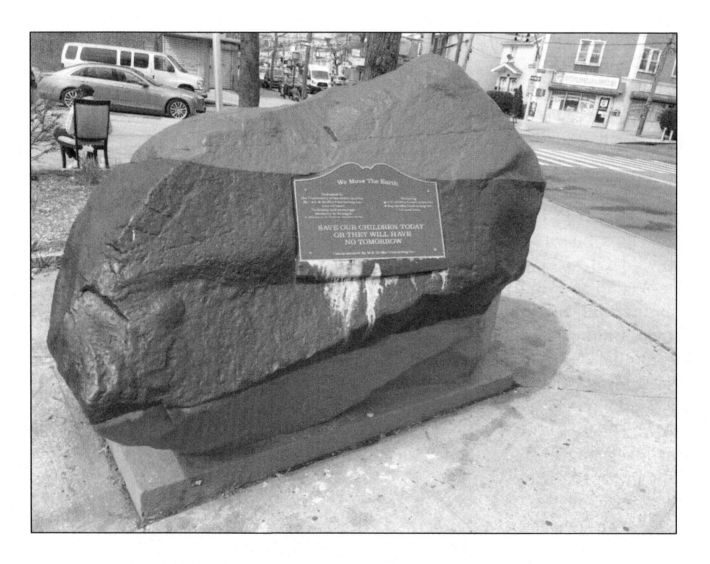

The Rock on Farmers Blvd. in Queens, New York!

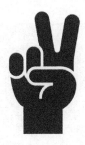

A Wonderful Omen

P.S. 118 is the first school I ever attended as a kindergarten student. My teacher was Mrs. Phillips. There was an incredible twist of fate involving one of our opening day parade grand marshals, former WOR-TV news anchor, and current Manhattan restaurateur Julian Phillips. Julian and I became friends attending the Christian Cultural Center in Brooklyn, New York. After the very spirited parade, we arrived at the landing spot, P.S. 118. Grand Marshal Julian Phillips had a "déjà vu" moment. Julian says to me, "Hey Hosea. I think I have been here before.

What's the name of this school?" "P.S. 118. I am the dean here," I said. "Man, can you believe that my mother used to teach kindergarten at this school," Julian said excitedly! "Wow. That is incredible! Brother, you will not believe this. Your mother was MY kindergarten teacher," I claimed! Just one of many serendipitous occurrences in my life. Please allow me to share my spiritual side with you. I call those incidents "God moments." To me, that is when the Lord is letting me know that something special is happening. I will dedicate a chapter to my God moments in my next book.

On those parade days, I had an acute sense of being aligned with my calling. Being spiritually connected to my purpose. My inspiring others to get involved. And some of the most significant people in basketball or sports, in general, are the mighty coaches!

ADVICE: Eliminate toxic people if they are creating a disruptive environment! Although it is a volunteer organization, it does not mean you have to subject the people you engage or yourself to abusive people. Sometimes you may have to make tough decisions.

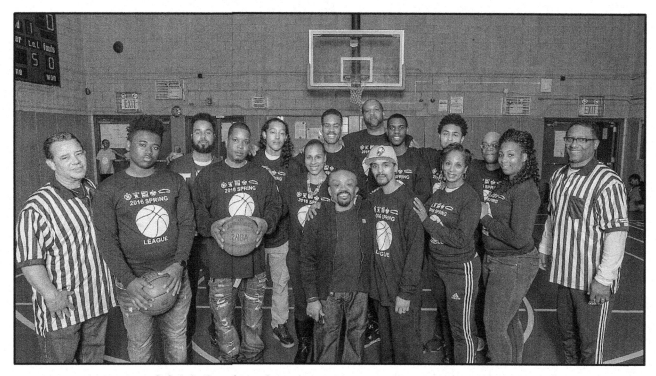

2016 Spring League (Photo credit - Erskine Isaac)

Starting Your Sports Program: 4 Things to Consider

1. Determine if it will be a club or a 501c3 nonprofit organization.
   - A 501C3 certification from the IRS allows donors to write off their contribution. A club has a much less formal structure and accountability requirements.

2. Do a name search. The process varies from state to state. Check with your state's department of state. For NYS submit a written request to the Department of State, Division of Corporations, One Commerce Plaza, 99 Washington Avenue, Albany, NY 12231.

3. Secure a tax id # (a.k.a. EIN #). You need this to open up a bank account.
   - https://www.irs.gov/businesses/small-businesses-self-employed/apply-for-an-employer-identification-number-ein-online

4. Identify a strong bookkeeper/treasurer or buy QuickBooks software for efficient record keeping.

Chapter 4

The COACH Project™
(Challenging Our Adults to Choose Helping)

"If we only had more soldiers, more battles would have been won and more lives would have been saved!"
~Anonymous Warrior

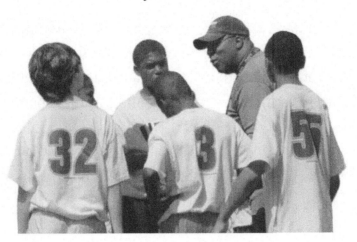

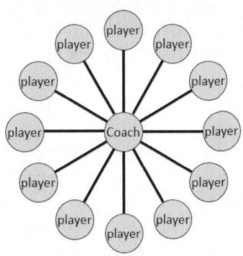

A mentorship ratio that empowers!

2coachateam.org

This project is designed to link adults who desire to coach with leagues across the country.

Many essential facets must be in place in order to be triumphant in developing a successful sports league. None is more important than having a solid coaching unit. Coaches are the heart and soul of any sports league. Coaches sacrifice their time and often their personal resources to help develop their players.

The ultimate goal of any sporting event is to win, to outscore your opponent by the end of the game. Winning the game is usually the measure of success for most coaches in most leagues. However, in addition to creating a team that wins games on the field or court, the best coaches are also training their players to be productive men and women in society, winning in the game of life.

Coaches hopefully understand the power they possess in shaping the hearts and minds of their players. Coaches have the capacity to reinforce in their players tools necessary for them to have meaningful and fruitful lives. In so many cases, a coach becomes a surrogate father or mother, specifically as it relates to Black and Latino urban male youth.

That's an enormous responsibility. A coach must mentally and emotionally prepare to accept the task. The coach is that role model that could help a young male understand the challenges he will face as he advances towards manhood.

It is important to note that being a role model doesn't mean one has had a perfect life. Sometimes, based on personal setbacks in life, some men and women feel no longer qualified to be an example for young people. The truth of the matter is that person who has overcome something and is striving to overcome challenges may be precisely what young people need to see, real-life experiences.

It's sad to say that the hyper-dysfunction of our inner-city communities is often perpetuated from generation to generation. In those situations, there is no clear blueprint for changing one's station in life. Coaches must understand that they have the power to alter a child's destiny. That's why the training of the coaches is vitally important. And picking good ones is just as crucial. Here are just a few fine examples of three coaches who are on the frontline. I will focus on three coaches I worked with within the South Bronx between 2012 through 2020, Coach G, Coach Tre, and Coach McKay. In my various roles, I have worked with, supervised, or coached against hundreds of coaches. However, I selected these three specific community coaches to highlight the challenges involving inner-city coaches in today's world. Each coach had significant character traits that were essential in building a sports league. It's critical to provide encouragement and support to the coaches, for they are the true change agents.

"No judgments within our domain. If you come into our gym with a true spirit and with pure intent to help our kids, all we see is a halo over your head."
~Hosea James Givan II

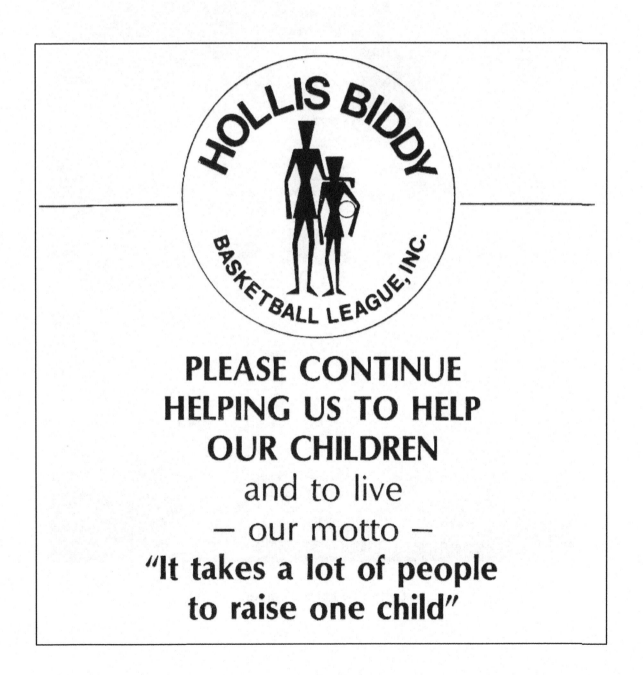

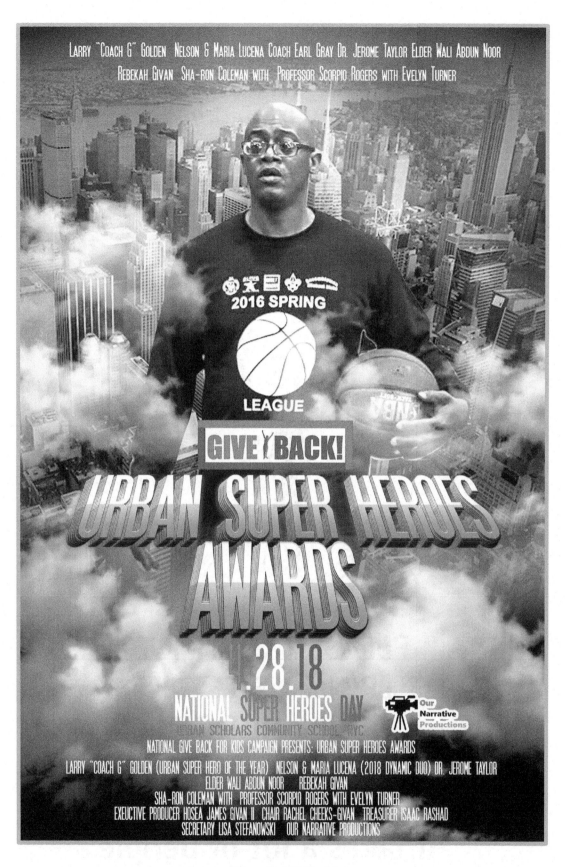

Larry "Coach G" Golden

Character Traits: Leadership and Loyalty

"A true soldier! As the battles raged on, he NEVER left his post!"
~ Hosea James Givan II

| Coach G |

Every day during school dismissal at P.S. 463 in the South Bronx, I was assigned to our schoolyard to monitor parents picking up their child or children. And every day at dismissal, I noticed a bald-headed, bespectacled, muscular Black man picking up his son. He was always on time and always looked serious and "about business," not the smiley type at all!

As we became more familiar with each other, we would engage in small talk as he waited for his son's class to join us in the schoolyard. The more we talked, the more I was impressed with this father by the name of Larry Golden.

His son, Khalid, was the nicest kid you will ever meet! He wore glasses like his dad and was a much skinnier version of his dad. Khalid was scholarly and always well-behaved.

Larry was a married father of three sons who lived three blocks from the school. He was a hardworking man, a contractor by profession, and brilliant, having skipped grades twice in elementary school. What really made me feel a connection to him was the fact that he was very civic-minded.

When I first created the Alpha Eagles Boys Club in partnership with the Bronx Alphas and the National Give Back for Kids Campaign in 2012, Larry Golden was the first parent-volunteer I recruited. My instincts about Larry were spot on. I based my hunch mainly on the way I saw him interact with his son.

As a volunteer, Larry always showed up, always on time, and took his role with the utmost seriousness. In addition, Larry connected well with the Alpha brothers. He even anointed himself an honorary Alpha and wore the black and yellow Alpha Eagle t-shirt (given to all the children and volunteers) with enormous pride. On occasion, Larry would boastfully shout, "0-6," something Alpha Brothers enthusiastically say to each other, usually as a greeting, in remembrance of the year the organization was founded (1906), at Cornell University in Ithaca, New York.

Before each Saturday morning session Larry Golden, who became affectionately known as "Coach G" and was beloved by the kids, conducted stretching exercises in a drill sergeant-like manner. Our young men genuinely appreciated his disciplined and no-nonsense mindset. Just about every Saturday, they also received a mini-sermon from him on the importance of academic excellence, concluded by reminding the young men that we will be checking grades! Despite that stern demeanor, his love for our boys radiated throughout the building.

The inaugural first year (2012) in the Bronx was terrific! Strong support came from the Alphas and was highlighted by a basketball clinic orchestrated by our legendary frat brother, Nate "Tiny' Archibald.

In Year Three (2014) of the Alpha Eagles Boys Club, we shifted our base of operations to the South East Bronx Neighborhood Center (SEBNC) at the edge of Forest Projects, located four blocks from P.S. 463. We were temporarily displaced as the gym was being renovated on the weekends, and the building was off-limits. The SEBNC was across the street from Golden's residence.

The volunteer support had radically scaled down from the two years before, but Coach G, occasionally one or two volunteers and I, helped keep things going. One of those volunteers became a part of our team. His name is Wali Abdun-Noor. As I think about it, we joined his squad!

> "He was the ultimate overcomer. He was trying his best to prevent our young men from making the same mistakes he had made. And for him, the whole experience probably was cathartic."

Wali Abdun-Noor, who I respectfully call "Elder Wali," was a bearded, army green hat-wearing septuagenarian who lived up the block from P.S. 463. We met one Saturday while at the SEBNC. He had heard about the things we were doing at the school and expressed appreciation for our efforts. Elder Wali was the epitome of a community servant and wore several civic-related hats. The one that was most relevant to our program was the one he wore running the local Boy Scout Troop 777 out of the SEBNC.

By the end of year three, the Alpha Eagles Boys' Club had morphed into the newly formed Boy Scout Troop 3777, and the Saturday program was back at P.S. 463. Although the gym was not yet finished, we utilized classrooms, hallways, and the teacher's lounge to conduct our activities. The ever adaptable and incredibly loyal Coach G was now one of the Boy Scout troop leaders, and the club had, for the time being, made a significant pivot away from basketball and life skills training into scouting. With the addition of a recently retired teacher from the school, bongo-playing Nelson Lucena, and his wife Maria, we continued to make Saturdays fun for our boys.

Year Four was a biggie. The new gym at P.S. 463 had finally been rebuilt! Each Saturday, the energy level and excitement were high. Between the Alpha Eagles Boys Club and basketball, we had upwards of 40 to 50 young men each week under our leadership. In that same year, Coach G shared with us during one of our discussions with the boys a part of his life he deeply regretted.

We learned that he had served time upstate in prison. He attributed that personal setback to being a follower and not a leader. That revelation explained why he had emerged into such a dynamic leader. It was a matter of survival. Through the years, he always emphasized to our young men, "Be a leader, not a follower!" Now we knew why. His brutal transparency made us love him even more! He was the ultimate overcomer. He was desperately trying his best to prevent our young men from making the same mistakes he had made. And for him, the whole experience probably was cathartic.

Coach G had evolved into the father of the neighborhood. His community ties allowed us always to keep close tabs on our boys. If he saw them in the street engaging in inappropriate behavior, he would "check" them. Due to the love and respect he had earned by his consistent caring through the years; they would adhere to his reprimand and fall in line. His passion and dedication had become contagious as we eventually attracted other strong fathers and mothers into our program.

In the spring of that fourth year, Coach G's coaching talents were on display as we formed the first Spring League Basketball Tournament. I was not surprised to discover that he was an outstanding coach! He was a skilled motivator and did a marvelous job of creating a family-like bond within his team. Maintaining his drill sergeant's toughness, he pushed his players to give their best effort. Just as he had done for the program, he poured his heart into his team, and consequently, they were winners!

April 28, 2018, the National Give Back for Kids Campaign created an opportunity to pay tribute to our most dedicated volunteer, Larry "Coach G" Golden. I learned that every year on April 28th, it was National Superhero Day. I am delighted to say that day also happens to be my birthday. With the knowledge of the significance of the day, we launched our first Urban Superhero Awards.

We identified ten people who had gone above and beyond to make a difference in our communities. We deservedly named Coach G our "Urban Superhero of the Year!" We celebrated his rise as a community leader. He was a dedicated father and husband. He used his experience in jail as a motivating force to make a positive impact on our youth.

We took advantage of his animated and high-energy personality on a couple of occasions and put him in the role of community spokesperson. He twice appeared on our weekly BronxNet cable show "IGNITE! EMPOWER! TRANSFORM!" He was that role model the community needed to know. We wanted to raise his visibility, and we did!

By 2020, our Saturday program, in addition to the Alpha Eagles Boys Club and basketball program, was comprised of both archery and tap dancing. We also had girls in the program. Things took a drastic change because of the Covid-19 pandemic. We are currently on hiatus until the Coronavirus reaches herd immunity, and we can resume our activities. However, there is one thing we know for sure. When we once again open the doors to the program, God-willing Coach G will be there! He's the rock you build a program around!

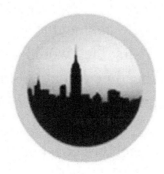

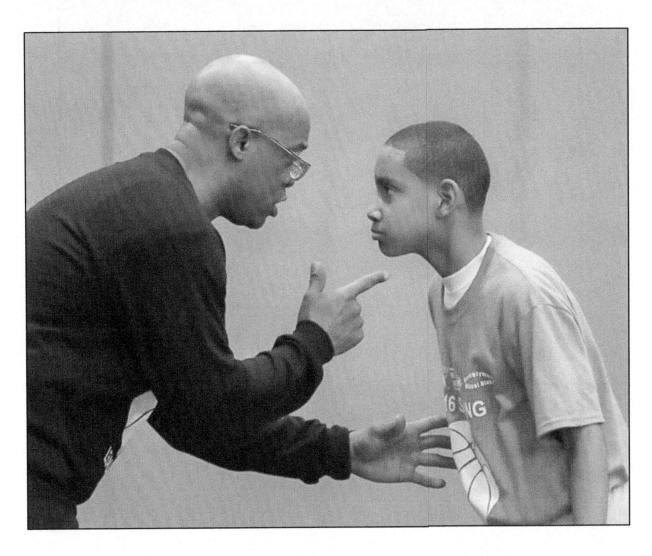

Coaches can instill discipline in their players.

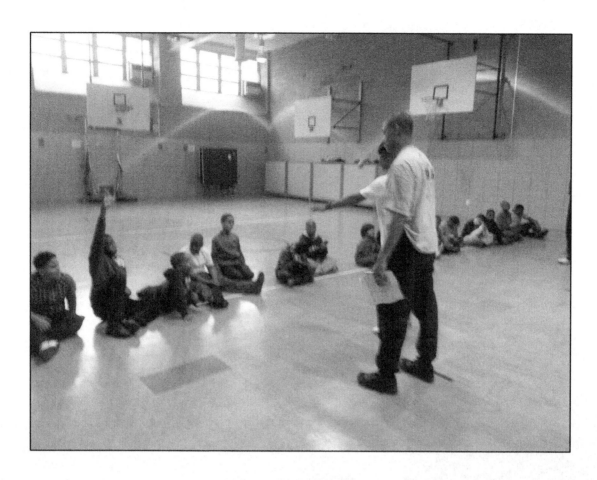

The Old Gym

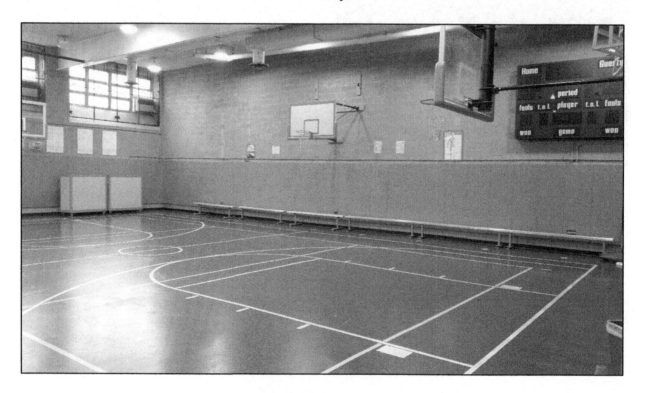

The New Gym

Character Traits: Punctuality and Reliability

| Coach Tre |

Tre McMillan is the father of one of my most challenging former students, Bryce. Although Bryce was a very bright student, his aggressive and defiant attitude constantly landed him in trouble. He seemed to have a permanent "chip on his shoulder."

I ran a basketball club at my school (P.S. 463) during the day on Tuesdays after the lunch period. During that time, I noticed that Bryce was pretty athletic and loved to play basketball. I stored that information.

As Bryce's guidance counselor, when a situation occurred and intervention was required, it often needed a "sit down" with his father. Tre McMillan is a wide-shouldered, 6-6, and 260-pound man. He has a charming personality and was always respectful. Tre is an old-school type of parent and did not blame "the system" for flaws in his son's behavior. He listened and tried to understand. He sometimes appeared overwhelmed by the challenges his son presented. Add to the mix a bit of "Baby Mama Drama" that seemed to creep into their lives from time to time. Nonetheless, McMillan never shirked his responsibilities and never blamed the school. Unfortunately, that is something some parents unjustifiably often did.

At the outset of forming the basketball league at my school, the second parent I contacted to coach in the league was Tre McMillan. He gladly accepted the offer, and we both felt the program would be excellent for his son. He also saw it as a bonding opportunity for Bryce and him.

When the league started, Coach Tre was unemployed. He lived on the block next to the school. I often saw him hanging out there as I drove through. He lived with his grandmother in the house where he grew up. Immensely popular around the school's parameters, Tre was one of the people that ingratiated me with his community. His neighbor Elder Wali, who I previously mentioned, was the other friendly neighbor.

Coach Tre was usually the first adult in the building on Saturdays. He waited patiently, just inside the door of the school, until I arrived. He loved interacting with the kids, playing ball with them, or just participating in the talks we often had with them. He graciously embraced the highly regarded title of "Coach." He was the first to start calling me "Commish," short for commissioner (of the league). Soon afterward, all the coaches referred to me in that way. I must say, I enjoyed that title.

He talked to me about how good it felt walking into a bodega, and one of the players would say, "Hey there, coach!" It really filled him with a sense of pride and increased responsibility to set a better example for his son and the neighborhood's young men. Moreover, like Coach G, he was able to redirect some of our guys if he saw them going down the wrong path. The operative word in that last sentence is "some." In managing expectations, I always let the coaches know that our goal was to save all our young people, but realistically, that will not happen. In this war for the hearts and minds of our youth, unfortunately, there will be casualties.

I saw a significant transformation in Tre those first two years. He began talking about taking civil service exams. I saw Tre less and less on the block. He was growing as a person and was aspiring for greater things in life. Nowadays, Tre consistently stays employed in construction-related jobs. He talks of becoming an electrician.

He recently credited me for being supportive and a positive influence in his life. For me, it was important not to be judgmental. I expected and allowed room for growth, but I always tried to be subtle in making my thoughts known as they pertained to "grown man things."

I cannot say what was going on in the block before I saw changes. At this point, I do not care. I can say Tre has proven to be highly dependable, and I am so thankful that he is an early riser! Sometimes, in creating a youth program, it is not only the children you affect. Some adults need that same kind of support and encouragement. So be mindful as you reach your community through basketball and sports programs that you are not just touching the lives of children. Coach G is an example of that, as well as Coach Tre. Next, I'll give you a glimpse at how a basketball or sports program can influence not just an individual adult or young person but an entire family.

The Hollis Biddy Basketball League's motto **"It takes a lot of people to raise one child,"** was derived from the African proverb

"It takes a village to raise a child." It appears that the saying originated from *Zulu's Ubuntu Philosophy*. Ubuntu is often translated as **"I am because we are!"** It is a concept that promotes the value of a supportive community working together for the benefit of all. (5)

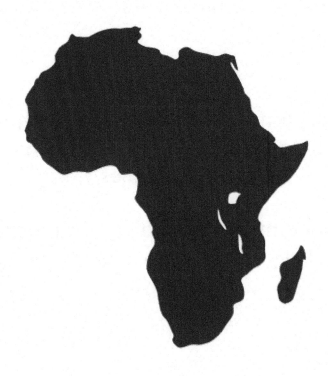

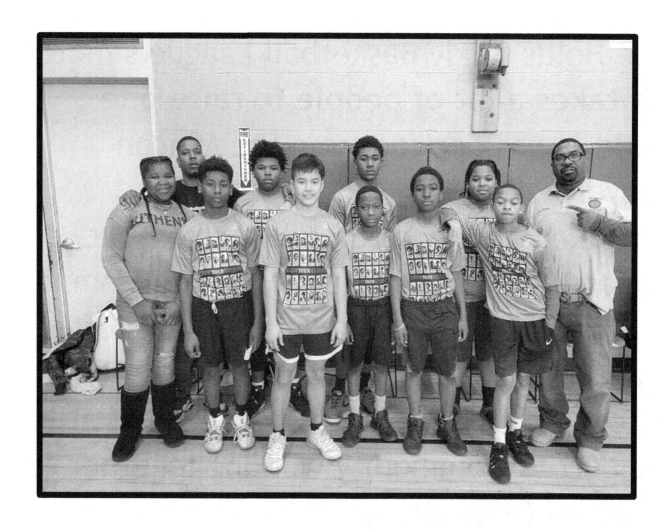

Boston 2020

"I told myself if I ever made it to the level
I want to be at, I'm gonna give back."
~LeBron James

"The most important thing is to try and inspire people so
that they can be great at whatever they want to do."
~Kobe Bryant

Character Traits: Tenacity and Resiliency

| Coach McKay |

Fred McKay was a coaching genius! His undefeated Cavaliers team had an equal balance of solid coaching and talented players that performed well under pressure. With his strong personality, he imposed his will on the court. And much to the chagrin of some, at times intimidated referees. He never went too far, though. I have no recollection of him ever receiving a technical foul. However, he did just enough to gain a favorable call or two later in the game.

McKay's gamesmanship was quite impressive. It was clear he understood psychology. He was cerebral in his approach to the game, sprinkled with high intensity. He held practice with his players on Saturdays (after the program) on the courts outside the school. The following week, his team was prepared, confident, and ready to take on their opponent.

McKay's son, Bristan, was a top player in the league. He was a natural shooter, and despite being a couple of years younger than some of the better players, he was fearless. Bristan was also an honor roll student at P.S. 463. He was never a problem, always focused and well-mannered. His mom, Kristan, was always at the games, coaching and rooting from the bleachers. Her oldest son Wally, from another relationship, was Coach McKay's assistant.

When the season ended, I encouraged Coach McKay to identify the best players in the league, form a team, and enter them in local summer tournaments. He took my advice and had the young men playing in two tournaments, one in the Bronx and the other at the Rucker Park in Harlem.

Like Coach Tre, Coach McKay grew up on the block next to the school. And like Coach Tre, Coach McKay was also raised by his grandmother. Tre and Fred have known each other their entire lives. Another common denominator Coach McKay shared with Coach Tre was that McKay was not working when I first met him and was often seen on the block or around the corner, just hanging out.

Like Tre, Fred was another coach who really benefitted from a heightened community status as a basketball coach. More importantly, his entire family loved his newfound greater community relevance.

It was such great news when McKay came and told me he got a job moving cars at a parking garage in Manhattan. Fred and his family were living in temporary housing and, at one time, commuted back and forth from Brooklyn to the Bronx. No small feat because of the distance. Regardless, Bristan and his younger sister stayed enrolled at P.S. 463. And, of course, Fred remained a coach.

I arranged for the family to visit a college-prep boarding school in northern Connecticut. It was an excellent opportunity for Bristan, who I felt would thrive in such an environment as a scholar-athlete. Upon visiting the campus, they were mesmerized by the beauty of the campus. After talking with my contact, I heard that the visit went well. I knew how important it was for families to be exposed to such opportunities. Not wanting this to sound like a cliché, but that experience truly broadened their horizons.

I set up other opportunities for the family to explore different experiences. They enjoyed luxury box seats at a Yankees game. The family attended a University of Connecticut men's basketball game. And Kristan was one of the featured speakers at the National Give Back for Kids Campaign's 10-Year Gala in Westchester, New York. Exposure to new things is so significant when trying to improve families' growth potential in our communities. We can go from one level to the next when possibilities can become realities.

Fred, who had never finished high school, was suddenly considering getting his GED and then planning to attend Bronx Community College. He had already spoken to one of my fraternity brothers, who was an administrator there.

"One day Kristan caught me in the main office on a school day and pulled me to the side, and said, 'Mr. Givan, you just don't know how much you have done for our family. Thank you!' I was

over the moon delighted to know that 'The Village' was making a difference."

Fred was eager and ready to improve the quality of life for his family and himself. Then, unfortunately, things started to unravel. He lost his job. He got caught up in a legal situation that wound up in court. But thankfully, Fred's case was thrown out. Things went from bad to worse when his grandmother (the woman that raised him) died. They were extremely close, and the loss impacted him greatly. At the wake, I met Fred's father for the first time. He was temporarily released from prison to attend his mother's funeral. He was in handcuffs and had shackles around his ankles. That sight helped me piece some things together.

Later that year (2019), Fred and I attended a free Brooklyn Nets coaching clinic at the Barclay Center. I marveled at how excited he was and watched him soak up all the basketball knowledge shared that evening.. It was a great clinic conducted by the Brooklyn Nets' coaching staff. During the trip, Fred opened up and confided in me like never before. I sensed a high level of trust. After four years of interacting with one another weekly (sometimes daily), that breakthrough moment finally occurred. Once again, I was witnessing growth.

Shortly after that, however, Fred and Kristan broke up. Of all the recent blows, this was the most devastating. Fred was a good father who loved his kids. Being separated from them would surely take its toll.

Sensing Fred was slipping away, I made a pitch to him. I offered him a chance to coach a team with our younger Saturday program kids at a 2020 Black History Month tournament in Boston. Bristan, having a birthday late in the year, was eligible to play. He jumped at the opportunity. For me, it was one more chance to keep him on a positive path.

We went up to Boston with two teams. A younger team from the Bronx (Morrisania Magic) and an older Hollis Biddies team coached by Charles Thomas.

At the tournament in Boston, I gave a presentation to all the teams about the "Importance of Giving Back," highlighted by our Give Back video. I also did an impromptu Black History Month presentation that went over well.

The trip was a success, although our boys did not do well. Bristan got to play on both teams, which was an excellent experience for him. The older kids did much better than the younger group. Overall, the players loved the trip to "The City on a Hill."

Before we left Boston, I had the teams make a pilgrimage our teams have been doing for more than 15 years. Our teams visited the Roxbury home of Malcolm X. While there, for the first time, we met Malcolm X's younger cousin, who came outside and talked to us. For Fred, that part of the trip was profoundly moving and left a lasting impression. When we returned to New York City, he expressed his gratitude for the experience. He was feeling good, and I was confident that he would follow through with the GED program and then go on to Bronx Community College. Two weeks later, New York City (like the rest of the world) was shut down due to the Coronavirus.

"I take Fred's potential ascension personally. He is so typical of too many Black men on the cusp of 40 years of age, in need of a breakthrough. Fred's brilliance has never been realized. I know it is there."

That summer, a chance for Bristan to attend a private school in Westchester came my way. I tried to reach Fred and Kristan for several months, leaving messages with family and friends. In December, I finally made a connection. However, the opportunity had passed.

There was an eight-month gap between the last time I had spoken to Fred and the time we reconnected. I was happy to hear the positive energy in his voice. I know he must have gone through a storm, but there was no such detection as I carefully listened. I remain optimistic. I take Fred's potential ascension personally. He is so typical of too many Black men on the cusp of 40 years of age, in need of a breakthrough. Fred's brilliance has never been realized. I know it is there. I had witnessed it several times in different situations. His ability to turn his life around could inspire many others. Like Tre, Fred was extremely popular in the Morrisania (South Bronx) community. His story is still unfolding, indeed a work in progress.

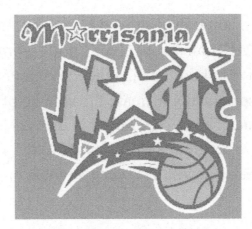

Morrisania Magic Logo

Caring coaches take a bow!

A coach that cares is elevated to an incredibly significant status in every inner-city community. Mind you, I did not say a winning coach, but a caring coach. A coach must be able to effectively convey to his or her players that they are not just interested in winning the game. More importantly, that coach needs to be concerned about the wellbeing and personal development of that player. When that caring coach walks into a local bodega, or what we used to call "Candy Store," and is identified by a player or parent, that coach is greeted with the highest sense of honor and respect.

In many cases, coaches never envisioned themselves being on such a high plateau. It may give them a sense of importance that they never felt before, filling a deep void. I mentioned earlier in the book that you sometimes never get to experience the feeling of reward for volunteer services rendered. Yet sometimes you do. The sense of pride associated with being identified as a community leader is truly rewarding for a job well done. That is the positive and transformative energy upon which a community can undoubtedly build. Preparing the coach to understand their power is also very crucial. They must be taught to manage their influence with grace and dignity.

The National Give Back for Kids Campaign has developed a solid 6-hour training program for coaches. However, we encourage our coaches to continue to seek further knowledge. My dear friend and Alpha Phi Alpha Fraternity brother, Coach Ted Gustus, has a solid training program through his "One Breath" initiative. The Positive Coaching Alliance is also another excellent resource for coaches. Contact information on both entities can be found in this book's appendix section and is filled with lots of invaluable forms and information to get you off to a great start.

I started this chapter highlighting The National Give Back for Kids Campaign's *The C.O.A.C.H. Project*. C.O.A.C.H. is an acronym for **Challenging Our Adults to Choose Helping.** I created the initiative to boost the number of volunteer coaches throughout the world. Its primary goal is to specifically increase the volume of inner-city community coaches in Black and Latino neighborhoods. Multiply the coaches coaching in community centers, P.A.L. centers, summer leagues, YMCA leagues, etc. The salvation of our inner-city youth could hang in the balance with the success of this program and similar programs.

We want to encourage men and women to connect with young people when they are still developing and very impressionable. We believe that coaches are a significant part of the solution towards healing and transforming inner-city communities. As I close this chapter, I leave you with the slogan of our C.O.A.C.H. Project as a reminder of why you should reach your community through basketball and other sports programs**.**

"Young people can't play on a team if they don't have a coach!"
~ Hosea James Givan II

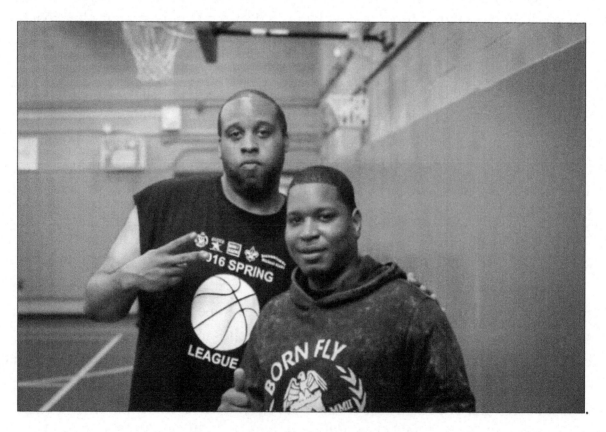

Coach Tre and Coach Fred

Preparing Athletes for Life After Sports

Through the years, I constantly had conversations with my players about building skill sets that would allow them to manage grown-up situations. We've talked about:

- The importance of good credit and paying your bills on time.

- The value of setting realistic short-term and long-term goals.

- The significance of choosing friends that enhance your life.

- The relevance of keeping your word and being honest.

- How toxic relationships can derail your life.

- Establishing a personal budget and living within your means.

Coaches utilize that down to time to enlighten your captive audience about important life lessons. Let your players know that there are support systems available to assist them with life after sports:

Continuing Education
http://www.acces.nysed.gov/bpss/welcome-career-training-proprietary-schools

Career Training programs
Year Up program https://www.yearup.org/students
Workforce 1 https://www1.nyc.gov/site/sbs/careers/careers.page

CUNY Initiatives (Including the Black Male initiative)
https://www.cuny.edu/academics/current-initiatives/
Work Training. https://bwiny.org/made-in-ny-pa-training-program/overview/

Social Services Programs
The Fatherhood project: https://www.thefatherhoodproject.org/teen-dads-forgotten-parent/

Young fathers resources
https://growingupnyc.cityofnewyork.us/generationnyc/topics/young-parents/
http://www.realdadsnetwork.org

Food Pantries.
https://www.foodpantries.org/

Mental Health and other resources for Teens https://www1.nyc.gov/site/doh/health/health-topics/teen-resources.page

World of Money
http://www.worldofmoney.org

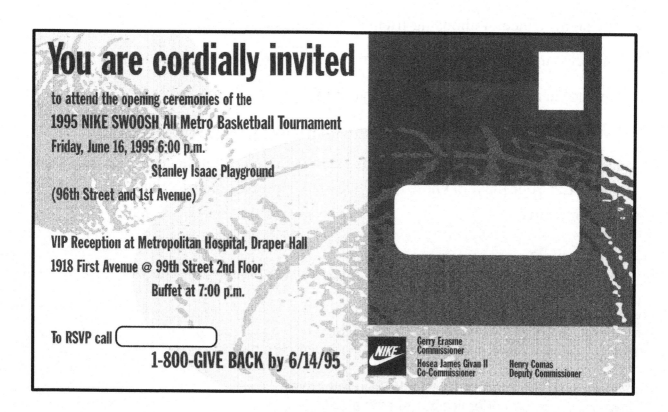

Nike Swoosh 1995

Epilogue

There are so many things causing strife and bitter discourse among human beings on Earth in the current state of the world. Sports can be the bridge to a better world. As evidenced by Nelson Mandela during South Africa's incredible 1995 Rugby World Cup Win, sports can have a socially transformative impact. In Mandela's own words, *"Sport has the power to change the world. It has the power to inspire. It has the power to unite people in a way that little else does. It speaks to youth in a language they understand. Sport can create hope where there was only despair."* (6)

Whether it is Eric Barnett, who runs both football and basketball programs in Queens, New York or Talib Yakini Reid, who leads a track and field program in Washington, DC or Veronica Vasquez, who ran that Parkchester Baseball Little League in The Bronx, New York; they all will testify to the beautiful ways their respective sport helps to develop our youth. I used the sport of basketball as my way to reach and inspire young people. However, hockey, soccer, swimming, or any other team sport can have the same effect upon our youth if appropriately presented.

Over the years, with the scores of young people I have coached, there was one message using my best "Jedi Mind Trick Technique" that I wanted every player always to remember, *"I have given to you. Your time will come to give back and when it does, do so."* League creators and coaches, please preach this message to your sports congregation. The world will change in miraculous ways as the spirit of giving back and helping others vibe grows stronger and stronger.

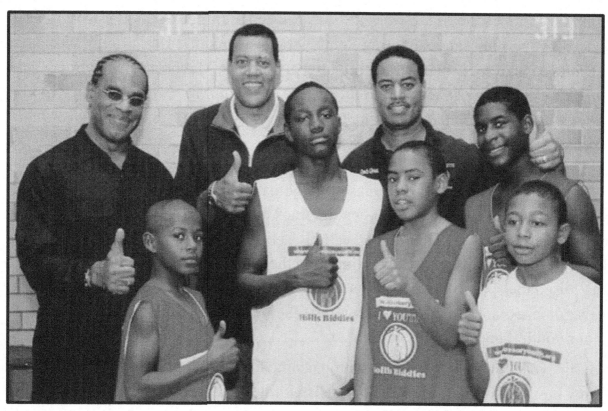

Judge Fred Sampson and Former NBA Executive V.P., Basketball Operations, Stu Jackson

Reach Your Community Through Basketball and Other Sports Programs

By Stu Jackson

Reach Your Community provided more than a "how-to" guide to positively affect communities using the universal language of sport. Hosea James Givan II's book provided us with motivation for how each of us can potentially impact young men's lives beyond the sporting games. Throughout the book, Hosea reinforces a need for community leadership and its thirst for positive role models. Hosea understands the far-reaching value mentors provide communities. Like the community role models he inspires, he has the ability to teach young people important life skills using basketball to encourage the many facets of the team concept. The lessons taught help them value their roles, the benefits of playing, and a sustained commitment for the greater good.

Givan helps readers understand whether we choose to coach or play; basketball is a privilege that can yield many ancillary benefits in the form of personal RECEIPTS for all involved. Many of these game receipts have lifelong positive effects on young players' lives, most of whom do not have the opportunity to make basketball a career or profession. Cases in point, Elijah McNeely, the game motivated him to improve academically and join a fraternity. Oswald R. Stubbs started out playing basketball at an early age only to realize his talent lay elsewhere. So he became a head coach when he turned 15 and later the Deputy Commissioner of the Hollies Biddies Basketball League (HBBL) at the age of 20. Charles Laws changed his early years of disruptive behavior. He also made a commitment to schoolwork after being rewarded with playing the game he loved. His turnabout was a direct result of having a presence of positive role models providing direction. Charles's life stabilized on a path that may not otherwise have been. In turn, Charles produced his own receipt sent to Hosea, his mentor: "I never got to thank you for the opportunities you gave me and for not quitting on me when everyone else did. I will forever be grateful and forever love you for that."

Hosea has been receiving and issuing receipts in the name of youth and community empowerment for most of his life. I became the beneficiary of one of those receipts twenty years ago when Hosea asked me to give time to participate in a Hollis Biddies Basketball League program. As a player, collegiate, professional coach, NBA League executive, and collegiate administrator, I have received countless youth program organizers' requests to engage student-athletes. At times, I have been approached by self-anointed coaches and program administrators whose objectives are to benefit from young players' exploitation financially (e.g., representing and trafficking access to players on their behalf for high schools, prep schools, and colleges, and beyond). As I came to know Hosea and understand his life's purpose, I grew to understand his father's legacy and his commitment to making his life's work to benefit youth and the communities where they live through basketball.

Community leadership and basketball are in Hosea's DNA. The day I arrived at HBBL, I saw a thriving youth organization solely committed to the game's values and the mentorship of young people led by a community-oriented man paying forward rewards with services rendered. Since accepting Hosea's invitation to the program that day, I have observed his career work with great admiration knowing grassroots community leadership truly exists and is in capable hands.

Hosea's book culminated in years of commitment, experience, and program execution by galvanizing community leaders and resourcing like-minded volunteers. Hosea spoon feeds potential community sports activists "how to" recruit prospective players and coaches, source facilities, fundraise, and lays out a timetable.

He even provides specific, nuanced details on what type of people to look for, particularly in key roles like coaches, when he highlights the importance of balancing the goal of winning games with life lessons while making adjustments with kids based on their circumstances. Hosea's book leaves little to the imagination as he offers a thorough community-based plan on a platter. However, the primary impetus fueling the writing of "Reach Your Community" is to provide a community plan and opportunity and signal a CALL TO ACTION. It gives us all a chance to energize communities and ourselves by making a commitment to serve them. We can honor Hosea and this book following his lead by providing our time, resources, and sacrifice to unify communities and build a sense of pride for our youth and ourselves.

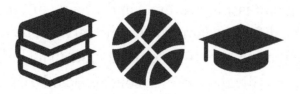

Community Coaching Opportunities

PAL	www.nationalpal.org
YMCA	www.ymca.net
JR. NBA	http://jr.nba.com
USA Basketball	www.usab.com
Boys and Girls Club of America	www.bgca.org
Amateur Athletic Union (AAU)	www.aausports.org
Reviving Baseball in Inner Cities (RBI)	www.mlb.com/rbi/
Soccer	www.usyouthsoccer.org
Football	http://playfoot.nfl.com/

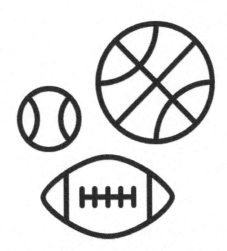

Foot Notes

1. James Naismith, Wikipedia, Wikimedia Foundation, https://en.wikipedia.org/wiki/James_Naismith
2. James Naismith, Wikipedia, Wikimedia Foundation, https://en.wikipedia.org/wiki/James_Naismith
3. The Importance of Promoting Diversity in Sports, The Sports Daily, https://thesportsdaily.com/the-importance-of-promoting-diversity-in-sport/
4. Amateur Athletic Union, Wikipedia Foundation, https://en.wikipedia.org/wiki/Amateur_Athletic_Union
5. Ubuntu Philosophy, Wikipedia, Wikimedia Foundation, https://en.wikipedia.org/wiki/Ubuntu_philosophy
6. Nelson Mandela, How Nelson Mandela used sport to transform South Africa's image, David Bond, https://www.bbc.com/sport/25262862

Photo Credits

1. Page 8 top (Hosea James Givan II)
2. Page 8 bottom (Hosea James Givan II}
3. Page 12 (Archives of Nate and Tena Archibald)
4. Page 16 (Givan Family archives)
5. Page 22 (Rucker Pro Legends Licensing)
6. Page 29 (Hosea James Givan II archives)
7. Page 32 (Erskine Isaac)
8. Page 37 (Hosea James Givan II archives)
9. Page 37 (Hosea James Givan II}
10. Page 39 (Hosea James Givan II archives}
11. Page 40 (Hosea James Givan II)
12. Page 48 {Hosea James Givan II archives}
13. Page 51 (Morgan Photography)
14. Page 52 top (Milton Carter, Jr.)
15. Page 52 bottom (Milton Carter, Jr.)
16. Page 56 (Hosea James Givan II)
17. Page 62 (James Coursey)
18. Page 64 (Erskine Isaac)
19. Page 65 (Hosea James Givan II)
20. Page 68 (Our Narrative Productions)
21. Page 72 (Erskine Isaac)
22. Page 74 top (Michael Givan)
23. Page 74 (Hosea James Givan II)
24. Page 78 (Hosea James Givan II)
25. Page 84 (Erskine Isaac)
26. Page 86 (Hosea James Givan II archives)
27. Page 88 (Milton Carter)
28. Page 21 (Hosea James Givan II archives)
29. Page 26 (Hosea James Givan II archives)
30. Page 28 (Hosea James Givan II archives)
31. Page 83 (Hosea James Givan II archives)

The quotations I used were gathered at times when I needed inspiration and hope. However, they were obtained unscientifically over several years or were contributed via family and friends. It's possible that the quotes are imperfectly worded or attributed. To the contributors, authors, and sources, THANK YOU and, where appropriate, my apology.

Covers designed by Oniel De La Cruz: onieldelacruz1@gmail.com

APPENDIX

The appendix is filled with lots of helpful documents
to help further you along your way.

Saturday Program
OPERATIONS MANUAL

Table of Contents

HISTORY

The National Give Back for Kids Campaign is a federally certified 501c3 not-for-profit organization created to motivate others to help our young people. Our primary inspiration was The Hollis Biddy Basketball League that is based in Queens, New York. In 1971, Hosea Givan, Sr. and Cecil Hollar, Jr. and several others, founded the program in an effort to present a positive alternative for boys and girls in Southeast Queens. After coaching two seasons in the East Harlem Biddy Basketball League, Hosea Givan, Sr. and Cecil Hollar, Jr., both IBM employees at the time, created the Queens program. They included not only a basketball league but also cheerleading and double-dutch programs as well, in order to offer both boys and girls an alternative to drugs and violence. The program was originally held at Andrew Jackson High School but soon moved to JHS 192. During this approximately 10-year phase of the Hollis Biddy Basketball League, over one thousand youngsters benefited from involvement with the league. The program was resurrected in 1994 and continues to impact lives in a positive way.

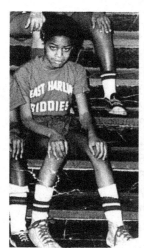

On June 2, 2009, Hosea J. Givan, II with the support of family and friends created the National Give Back for Kids Campaign. The organization has run a successful Saturday Program for children at P.S. 198 Campus in the Bronx. The program features life skills/leadership training, guest speakers, tap dance, basketball, and archery. The organization also hosts a weekly public access cable program, IGNITE! EMPOWER! TRANSFORM! The show highlights people making a difference in their communities. The organization hosts a second award winning show, "Bekah's Constellation" where young people a promoted for doing good work in their communities.

Another important project of the National Give Back for Kids Campaign is the annual Urban Superheroes Awards conducted every year on April 28th, National Superhero Day. On that day, the organization celebrates special individuals that go above and beyond to uplift their communities.

MISSION STATEMENT

The National Give Back for Kids Campaign, Inc. is a federally certified 501c3 non-profit organization dedicated to inspiring adults to "give back" through volunteering to work with children, recognizes that positive and substantial change can come about through the power of love and sacrifice; lives can be changed and communities empowered!

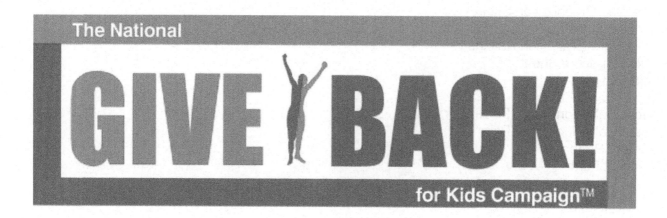

I. Board of Directors

The Name of Your Organization is primarily governed by its Board of Directors, which consists of seven volunteer members of varying abilities and professional experience. These voting members are:

Person A – Chair
Person B – Treasurer
Person C – Secretary
Person D – Member-at-large
Person E –Honorary Youth Member-at-large
Person F – Member-at-large
Person G – Member-at-large
Person H – Member-at-large
Person I – Member-at-large
Person J – Member-at-large

Chair – The Chair maintains overall responsibility of all The Name of Your Organization programs. The Chair is expected to foster relationships in an effort to leverage additional resources for programmatic and organizational activities. The Chair is the chief spokesperson for the organization. The Chair presides over the Board of Directors quarterly meetings and sets the meeting agenda in accordance with the organization's by-laws and constitution.

Treasurer – The treasurer maintains saving and checking accounts, summarizes income and expenses, files taxes, makes arrangements with the appropriate limited number of people to be authorized to make purchases for the programs, maintains a list of businesses where The Name of Your Organization's non-profit status has been registered, provides instructions for structuring purchases such that payments are made directly from NGBFKC bank accounts.

Secretary – The secretary monitors the post office box, maintains registration records, publicizes league upcoming meetings, records minutes of meetings, helps to maintain the website, coordinates league insurance coverage, assists desirable:

> Webmaster – Supervises www.TheNameofYourOrganization.org website.
> Saturday Program Registrar – Catalogs all incoming registration data.

Members-at-large – Assists in the strategic development and overall enhancement of the programs and organization. This includes advice and counsel, fundraising, program assessment, and risk management.

II. Executive Director

Executive Director – The Executive Director is the Chief Executive Officer of The Name of Your Organization. The Executive Director reports to the Board of Directors and is responsible for the organization's consistent achievement of its mission and financial objectives. In program development and administration, the Executive Director will:

Specific committee responsibilities:

1. Assure that the organization has a long-range strategy that achieves its mission, and toward which it makes consistent and timely progress.

2. Provide leadership in developing program, organizational and financial plans with the Board of Directors and staff and carry out plans and policies authorized by the board.

3. Promote active and board participation of volunteers in all areas of the organizational work.

4. Maintain official records and documents, and ensure compliance with federal, state, and local regulations.

5. Maintain a working knowledge of significant developments and trends in the field.

In communications, the Executive Director will:

1. See that the board is kept fully informed on the condition of the organization and all important factors influencing it.

2. Publicize the activities of the organization, its programs, and its goals.

3. Establish sound working relationships and cooperative arrangements with community groups and organizations.

4. Maintain official records and documents, and ensure compliance with federal, state, and local regulations.

5. Maintain a working knowledge of significant developments and trends in the field.

In relations to staff, the Executive Director will:

1. Be responsible for the recruitment, employment, and release of all personnel, both paid staff, and volunteers.

2. Ensure that job descriptions are developed, that regular performance evaluations are held, and that sound human resources practices are in place.

3. See that an effective management team, with appropriate provision for succession, is in place.

4. Encourage staff and volunteer development and education and assist program staff in relating their specialized work to the total program of the organization.

5. Maintain a climate that attracts, keeps, and motivates a diverse staff of top quality people.

In budget and finance, the Executive Director will:

1. Be responsible for developing and maintaining sound financial practices.

2. Work with the staff, Finance Committee, and the board in preparing the budget; see the organization operates within budget guidelines.
3. Ensure that adequate funds are available to permit the organization to carry out its work.

4. Jointly, with the president and secretary of the board of directors, conduct official correspondence of the organization, and jointly, with designated officers, execute legal documents.

Basketball League Checklist

- ☐ Create a budget.
- ☐ Identify a way to cover all expenses.
- ☐ Secure Liability Insurance.
- ☐ Lock in a site. Get the space agreement in writing.
- ☐ Promote the league via flyers, posters, social media and word of mouth.
- ☐ Identify coaches and table crew (Clock, Scoreboard, Official Scorebook and Stats).
- ☐ Screen and train all volunteers for their roles.
- ☐ Mandatory Sexual Abuse training.
- ☐ Register, measure height and rate the skill level of the young people for the league.
- ☐ Develop a fair selection process to create balanced teams.
- ☐ Order uniforms.
- ☐ Create a schedule for the season.
- ☐ Hire basketball officials (Highly recommended).
- ☐ Have a meeting reviewing the rules with the players, coaches and parents.
- ☐ Coaches meeting to reinforce expectations.
- ☐ Parade to engage the community.
- ☐ Start the league.
- ☐ Order trophies.
- ☐ Playoffs
- ☐ Create a fair system to identify special awards (i.e. MVP, Most Improved).
- ☐ Evaluate Coaches
- ☐ Awards ceremony. Disseminate info about the start date for the next season.

HJG2 2021

Recruitment

Volunteer recruitment is the process of attracting and inviting people to consider involvement with the organization. The Name of Your Organization is an organization that promotes loving and nurturing children. Therefore, we hope to attract volunteers with loving and nurturing personalities. The recruitment should identify people who both are warm and friendly and enjoy helping to develop strong children.

Recruitment Message
The recruitment message should be inviting and encourage people to become involved with your organization. The organization has multiple recruitment messages tailored to the volunteers being sought, such as students, professionals, neighborhood residents, past residents, and adults who benefited from youth programs as children.

Recruitment Strategies
The two most common strategies used to recruit volunteers for defined positions are *non-targeted* recruitment and *targeted* recruitment. Non-targeted recruitment means looking for people with general skills, such as volunteers to participate in security or fundraising. Targeted recruitment involves looking for people with specific skills, such as lawyers, coaches, or graphic artists. Both strategies must use the recruitment messages as described above.

Recruitment Process
People most often volunteer when they feel they are being asked to get involved personally. Don't assume a general advertisement in a newspaper or a public service announcement on the radio or TV will attract all or most of the volunteers you need. People need to be asked again and again! Recruit for specific projects and programs throughout the year rather than during a once-a-year campaign. When The Name of Your Organization is recruiting volunteers, it should involve the entire organization, from the CEO to the board of directors, or the clients to currently active volunteers. In addition, peers may be especially good at recruiting students and professionals.

Recruiting for Diversity
Diversity should be an essential element in your recruitment plan. In addition to race and ethnicity, consider other components of diversity, such as age, gender, education, income levels, religious beliefs, physical abilities, and skills. Know the demographics of the community your organization serves. The organization will be more effective if both your paid staff and your volunteer staff reflect the community it serves. This demonstrates to the community that people are assets, and it tells your consumers that you value them as partners, not just as clients.

Finally, consider deliberate and strategic outreach to youth, seniors, and people with disabilities. These groups have traditionally been viewed as targets of volunteer efforts, not as potential volunteers. Everyone has something to offer, and The Name of Your Organization may be in an ideal position to bring out the best in those who are rarely asked to volunteer.

Recruiting Techniques Used by the National Give Back for Kids Campaign, Inc.
There are many techniques available for recruiting volunteers. You must decide which is best for disseminating the recruitment message for your organization and your specific volunteer positions. The National Give Back for Kids Campaign, Inc. (NGBFKC) was created to provide grassroots urban organizations with assistance in the area of volunteer recruitment. In July 2012, NGBFKC launched the *Give Back Freedom Tour as a way to generate awareness for the urgent as to link volunteers with youth organizations.*

The campaign will be promoted through the following outlets:
* Mass media -- print and broadcast
* Public speaking
* Outreach to membership or professional organizations
* Multi-Media Presentations

- Music Videos
- PSAs
- Videotapes
- Direct mail
- Articles in local newspapers and newsletters of other organizations
- Referrals from individuals associated with your organization
- Flyers and Posters
- "Word-of-mouth"
- Volunteer fairs
- Internet web-sites
- Volunteer Center referrals

Retention

Understanding volunteers' motivations and remaining sensitive to their needs are essential to retaining volunteers. People's reasons for volunteering can differ dramatically. Regular and open communication will help determine the motivating element specific to each volunteer. Remember, also, that personal motivations can change over time.

Basic Motivation Factors

The Name of Your Organization has found four primary reasons why people choose to volunteer:

- Obligation: People, who have been the beneficiaries of volunteerism as youngsters, often have an intrinsic desire to "give back" and help others.
- Recognizing need: Volunteers are often motivated by a sense of mission to help change the current negative patterns in society.
- Achievement: A person motivated by achievement may seek to learn new skills through participation in a project.
- Affiliation/Socializing: In large part, these people volunteer because they enjoy the social aspects of the work. They often want to be identified as a person "who cares.

Assessing Motivation

The better you get to know a volunteer, the better you'll be able to identify that volunteer's motivation. Two-way communication is the key to success. Some strategies for keeping abreast of a volunteer's satisfaction include:

- Regularly sharing new developments in the program, the organization, and the field.
- Periodically soliciting the volunteer's suggestions about the program.
- Finding out what the volunteer likes most about her/his volunteer assignment and, if necessary, moving her/him to a position that includes more of what they enjoy.
  Another strategy for retaining volunteers is promoting exceptional volunteers to more responsible positions. Think of a volunteer "career path" within the organization. A volunteer for an event, for example, might be recruited to become a volunteer for a sustained position and eventually be placed on the board of directors. Again, ongoing and open communication will be the key to keeping volunteers engaged within the organization. For example, a newsletter to event volunteers will keep them informed of additional volunteer opportunities.

Volunteer Training

Coaches are expected to participate in six hours of training. General volunteers must go through a two-hour training session. New coaches will be connected with veteran coaches the first year to provide direct guidance and assistance. Training gives volunteers the direction, support and skills necessary to carry out assigned responsibilities. Training is typically provided by the staff in the area of the organization where the volunteer is assigned. In general, training should be:

- Giving volunteers a sociological insight into the population they are serving.
- Specific to the requirements of the volunteer position.
- Geared to the skill level of the volunteer.
- Training should be ongoing.
- Address needs to be identified by both volunteer and supervisor.
- Periodically evaluate to determine if training is on track.

Training is also a form of recognition and serves to keep a volunteer motivated, committed, and performing the quality of service you expect. Sending a volunteer to a special class or conference can be a reward for service, even if the class is not directly related to the volunteer's assignment but is of broad interest to your organization, such as CPR training, public speaking, conflict resolution, or team building.

Recognition
Recognition is how an organization tells volunteers that their efforts are important. Expressing thanks for donated time, energy, and expertise makes volunteers feel valued and appreciated. Praising individual volunteers, as well as the group, is a key volunteer retention strategy.

Recognition should be frequent and personal. Being sensitive to what volunteers expect helps the program administrator to design appropriate recognition activities. For example, volunteers seeking power may enjoy being thanked by the executive director and board of directors. A simple thank you from the paid staff may be appropriate for volunteers motivated by achievement. A party is right for the folks who volunteer to socialize.
Finally, even when a volunteer is satisfied with his or her position in your organization and is properly recognized, life events, such as family re-location, may require the volunteer to move on. Use the volunteer program continuation/termination policies to help plan for turnover among your volunteers.

Awards for Volunteer Service
The National Give Back for Kids Campaign's Urban Superhero Awards recognizes exemplary volunteers on National Superheroes Day, April 28th.

Screening

In any volunteer organization, the screening of volunteers is perhaps the most important function toward establishing a safe and stable environment for the children you will be servicing.

Each volunteer will be required to fill out an application. The application provides an area for two references and volunteer experience. Each reference must be thoroughly checked out. In addition, any volunteer directly interacting with children will be required to go through an interview process. A three-panel interview team will ask a series of questions to get a sense of the character of the volunteer. We recommend that each volunteer is fingerprinted to determine if there is any history of engaging in child abuse or violent criminal behavior.

There are several online services that can assist in doing background checks on potential volunteers. **Backgroundchecks.com** is one such organization. Through their service they are able to:

- Run a Personal Background Check
- Identify Sex Offenders
- Search State and National Criminal Records

Again, properly screening volunteers is essential in creating a volunteer staff of productive and effective givers. Historically, pedophiles gravitate to youth programs (i.e. Boy Scouts). Above all else, take every extra precaution to assure the safety of your children. **DO NOT PLACE A VOLUNTEER IN ANY TASK UNTIL THE ESSENTIAL RESEARCH ON THAT PERSON!**

Marketing

Flyer distribution is the primary means of marketing the program. Flyers are circulated in schools (with the permission of the Administration) and throughout the community (i.e. grocery stores, barbershops, hair salons, and libraries).

If an accurate database is kept from the previous year's enrollment, a postcard or email can be sent to potential participants to notify them about the program registration date. Our website also promotes the dates for registration.

Finally, the best advertisement for the program is a well-run, fun-filled program from year to year. If the participants and their parents are enjoying the experience, they will spread the news by telling, family, friends, neighbors, and co-workers about the effectiveness of the program.

Registration Process

The program is "first come, first serve." There is no "trying out." Enrollment is not based on talent or ability, but by an applicant simply registering before the deadline and/or before the program capacity is filled. Each registrant must be accompanied by a parent or guardian to sign the child up for the program. For many children, this will be their only opportunity to play on a team; a memory they will cherish for the rest of their lives.

The registration process should be well organized since this could be the family's first impression of the organization. Volunteers with good "people skills" and who conduct themselves with the highest level of professionalism should be performing the registration process. Good record keeping is vital and copies should be made of all applications. A set of the applications should be kept in a binder and be made available for all activities.

Student-Athlete Behavior Policy

1. Respect all adults.
2. Respect the other participants.
3. No fighting.
4. No profanity.
5. Participants can't roam the building alone. A child must be with an adult at all times.
6. Respect the building (i.e. bathrooms, bulletin boards, stairways).
7. Each week bring to the program the progress reports (school and home).
8. Come to the program each week with a clean uniform.

The Code of Behavior is to be reviewed initially with the player and their parent and letter collectively with the team and the coach. Each player will be required to sign the form acknowledging their understanding and acceptance of the code.

A violation of the code could result in the player being terminated from the program. The players are informed of this at the very outset of the program.

The Behavior Code will be reviewed every week for the first three weeks of the program.

Four Commitments

Each child will be expected to honor four commitments:

1. Get educated enough to establish a career or business.
2. When you're able to help others, GIVE BACK!
3. Be a good father (or mother) and be a good role model.
4. Maintain a healthy mind, body, and spirit.

Our commitments to them:

1. Each child in our program will feel loved and respected.
2. Each child will have an organization they will always belong to.
3. Each child will learn important things they may not learn in school.
4. We will do our best to prepare you for a leadership role in this world.

League Rules

1. <u>Divisions</u> - There will be two divisions: A) Next Level (Five teams, ages 10 through 12) and B) Future Stars (Four teams, ages seven through nine).

2. <u>Game Time</u> - Seven minutes running time for Next Level Division. Six minutes running time for Future Stars Division. The clock only stops for time-outs. Stop time last one minute of the 2nd and 4th quarters.

3. <u>Overtime Period</u> - First overtime period will be two minutes. If there is a second overtime period, the first team that scores will win.

4. <u>Uniforms</u> - Each player must wear an official league uniform. NO EXCEPTIONS! Replacement uniforms are available (Next Level $50 and Future Stars $10). Allow 7-10 days for delivery.

5. <u>S.C.O.P.E. Sheets</u> - Each player must submit S.C.O.P.E. sheets before the start of each game in order to play.

6. <u>Pressing</u> - No pressing in Future Stars Division. Pressing is allowed in the Next Level Division. If a team has a 15 point lead, no pressing is allowed by the team that is winning.

7. <u>Bathroom Usage</u> - Coaches or assistant coaches must escort their players to the bathroom. NO EXCEPTIONS!

8. <u>Play-offs</u> - There will be no play-offs. Standings will strictly be determined by the SCOPE System.

9. <u>Technical Fouls</u> - A player receiving a technical foul is suspended for one game. If a play receives a second foul, he is banned from the league. Coaches, who receive a technical foul, will be required to pay a $25 fine. The fine must be paid prior to the beginning of the next game.

10. <u>Second Quarter Rule</u> - The second quarter is designated for the "bench players." The least skilled players should be playing during the quarter. This has been a long-standing tradition in the Hollis Biddy Basketball League.

Team Selection Process

The players are selected in a "draft" scenario by the coaches. Each coach will choose in reverse order of the previous year's standings. The first place coach will choose and last and the last place coach will choose first. The coach is allowed two minutes in between draft selections. Each "round" will maintain the same order.

Draft Night is the night the coaches always look forward to. It's a night of fun, laughs, and good socializing. It has always been a night of bonding for the coaches. The Draft is usually conducted in the home of one of the coaches. Food and drinks add to the ambiance.

It is recommended that a neutral person is selected as the timekeeper and sergeant-of-arms; a coach can get deeply passionate about selecting his or her team!

The SCOPE Program

The S.C.O.P.E. Program was developed by Hosea James Givan II. It was modeled after the G.O.A.L.S. (Guaranteeing Options for Achieving Life Success) program instituted by the North Carolina YMCA Black Achievers Program and the Holland Holton Middle School of Durham. The program was designed to foster *improved academic performance* and *school citizenship*. GOALS was enhanced by Hosea James Givan II's SCOPE Program by creating a category that monitors *household chores* (i.e. taking out the garbage or cleaning one's bedroom) and by developing a more simplified rating system.

S.C.O.P.E. is an acronym that stands for *"School and Chores Optimizing Performance Evaluation."* Many young boys and girls today have dreams of becoming professional entertainers, and as parents and or concerned adults we should encourage our youth to dream. In reality, however, only few amounts will reach that "next level" in entertainment (i.e. The NBA or Hollywood). Nonetheless, the possibility of entering other professions or starting a business is quite good. The key to accessing these other career options is an educational achievement. Through educational achievement, students can optimize their opportunities for a successful professional career.

In the SCOPE Program, the boys and girls will be placed on teams that will compete in home chores recreational, and academic activities. The rationale for forming "teams" to improve school performance follows from research showing that for African American and Latino youngsters, the peer group exerts a strong influence over their academic value system. Even with strong school and parental support for academic activities, the African American and Latino peer group can sabotage these efforts by characterizing school achievers as "uncool," thus socially isolating them. It is also clear that for young African American and Latino boys and girls, participation in team activities builds brotherhood and sisterhood among team members. Therefore, our goal is to combine cooperation and competition with a team program that serves to improve performance in school (academics) and at home (chores). Thus, we optimize the chance of success in life for our children.

In the SCOPE Program, peer support for academic performance will be fostered by the common goal of having the "team win." At the same time, it is hoped that students will also establish new and more beneficial classroom and "home chore" habits.

Each boy and girl will have a weekly statistics sheet that will show his or her performance on activities associated with academics, school citizenship, and household chores.

League Standings

Regular basketball leagues base their standings on win/loss records. The SCOPE Program determines its team standings on program attendance, individual student performance in school and with home chores, and finally, the team win/loss record. The following criteria will be used to determine individual statistics and team standings:

1. **School Performance** - Players can receive up to five points (five being the highest, one being the lowest) for each of the following weekly activities: (a) Class attendance (b) Having work materials, including writing utensils, paper, and relevant books; (c) Classroom attentiveness; (d) Homework; and (e) Attitude.   It is each student's responsibility to ask his teacher to fill out and initial the rating form at the end of each week. A student can earn up to 25 points. For example:

Attended Class	**5**
Had Work Materials	**5**
Paid Attention	**5**
Homework	**5**
Attitude	**5**

Total = 25

2. **Household Chores** - Each week a player can also receive points by effectively doing his household chores. These points will be given based on the parents' assessment of their child's diligence in completing his chores.   Between one and five points can be earned in the "clean room" category. Another chore will be selected at the discretion of the parents. Finally, the category of behavior/attitude can earn the child another five points.

Based on 3 categories (2 chores and behavior) a child can earn up to 15 points, for example:

Cleaned Room	**5**
Took Out Garbage	**5**
Behavior/Attitude	**5**

Total = 15

3. **Fighting or Other Disruptive Behavior** - The students will have ten points subtracted for fighting or any other disruptive behavior in school.

4. **Disrespect to Parents or Siblings** - Any disrespect to parents and or siblings will cause a student to have five points subtracted from her score.

Point System

A team with 12 players can earn up to 480 points per week.

1. An average will be taken of the points each student-athlete. If each player gets 40 points, the team average will be **40 points (maximum amount).**   **Total team points ÷ # of players.**

> **For example: 400 ÷ 10 = 40**

2. If a team has at least 10 players in attendance it will receive 20 bonus points.

3. If the team wins their basketball game, it will receive **20 points** if 10 players are present. If the team wins with less than 10 players, it will only receive **0 points**. If a team loses their game it receives **10 points**. However, if the team loses the game **(10 points)** and has at least 10 players **(20 points),** it can receive **30 points,** thus outpointing a victorious team with less than 10 players **(20 points).**

> **Maximum points a team can earn:**
>
> **40 points, team average**
> **20 points for attendance**
> **10 for team basketball victory**
> **70 Total Team Points!!!**

Role of Coaches

The coaches for the individual teams are an integral part of the **SCOPE Program**. In addition to their basketball coaching duties, coaches are expected to play a mentorship role for their team members, which goes beyond the actual games. In particular, coaches are expected to review student point totals at the end of each week and provide reinforcement for areas where the students are excelling, and encouragement and guidance in those areas where they need improvement. Thus, it is the instructor's responsibility to guide the students in basketball, household, and academic activities.

Contract with Students

Students are required to sign a contract that outlines all of the goals and expectations of the program.

Travel Team Policy

Travel teams will be created by identifying the most talented players from the Saturday Program.

Each team must determine how the money will be raised to participate in prospective tournaments:

a. Elect a treasurer and create a budget
b. Plan fundraising events
c. Ensure financial viability
d. As these initiatives are outside the regular operating budget of The Name of Your Organization, there is no guarantee of money being available for individual teams choosing to participate in these tournaments.

Four fundraisers per year will be devoted to the travel teams:

a. Coaches Who Cook
b. Organization Gear Sales Drive
c. Alumni All-Star Game
d. Annual Alumni Solicitation Drive

Any monies raised through the fundraising efforts of the team will remain the property of the team. A separate banking account has been set up for each team. Any direct personal donations made to a specific team will remain with that team's account. For example, if a deposit amount is paid directly by the player (or parent) to the team, and that player does not go on the trip, that amount may be returned to the player. However, if the player participates in a team fundraising event (i.e. bottle drive, chocolate sales, etc.) any money raised in this way remains with the team. A team treasurer must be designated and provide an accounting of all monies when requested to do so by members of the team or by The Name of Your Organization. It is to each team's discretion whether they choose to offset costs for coaching staff traveling with the team.

Code of Conduct:
All teams must represent our organization and organization values at all times. (Please refer to the coaches, player and parent Code of Conduct Agreements signed prior to league play.) In addition, The Name of Your Organization asks the following:

Attire:
All players and coaching staff must wear sanctioned The Name of Your Organization Gear when playing, training, and otherwise representing our club as a team in any capacity. When traveling, especially internationally, it is advisable to wear The Name of Your Organization Gear for easy identification of team members. This The Name of Your Organization Gear must be regularly available The Name of Your Organization Gear, not any special order or special design items and in the standard The Name of Your Organization Gear colors.

Conduct:
All players, coaching staff and chaperones must represent our organization, our community and our City positively. All property and persons will be treated with respect. Coaching staff and chaperones will be held responsible for the behavior of the players. Any inappropriate incidents will result in evaluation and appropriate action from the Discipline Committee and may result in suspension of team travel and, in severe cases, the suspension of the person in question from The Name of Your Organization. The Name of Your Organization has worked hard to build relationships The Name of Your Organization to continue and increase participation in these programs. Therefore, our organization counts on each person to be a goodwill ambassador for The Name of Your Organization when traveling.

Alcohol, Drugs and Tobacco Policy

Alcohol, Drugs and Tobacco Policy The Name of Your Organization prohibits the use of alcoholic beverages and controlled substances at events of activities conducted by The Name of Your Organization or at any activity involving the participation of our youth members.

Adult staff or volunteers should support the attitude that young adults are better off without tobacco and may not allow the use of tobacco products at any The Name of Your Organization activity involving youth participants.

All The Name of Your Organization functions, meetings, and activities should be conducted on a smoke-free basis, with smoking areas located away from all participants.

Reporting Child Abuse

The following section outlines the guidelines from The Child Abuse Prevention and Treatment Act (CAPTA, 1996).

What counts as Child Abuse?

The minimum definitions for child abuse and neglect are any recent act or failure to act:
  a. Resulting in imminent risk of serious harm, death, serious physical or emotional harm, sexual abuse, or exploitation.
  b. Of a child (under 18 years of age)
  c. By a caretaker (teacher, babysitter, coach, etc.) or parent who is responsible for the child's welfare.

The minimum definitions for sexual abuse are:
  a. Employment, use, persuasion, inducement, enticement, or coercion of any child to engage in, or assist any other person to engage in any sexually explicit conduct or any simulation of such conduct for the purpose of producing any visual depiction of such conduct; or
  b. Rape, and in cases of the caretaker or inter-familial relationships, statutory rape, molestation, prostitution, or any other form of sexual exploitation of children, or incest of children.

The minimum definitions for emotional abuse are:
A sustained, repetitive pattern of behavior that demonstrably impairs a child's emotional development or sense of self-worth. This can include constant criticism, threats, rejection, or confinement, as well as withholding love, support or guidance.

The minimum definition for neglect is the failure to provide for a child's basic needs. Can include:
  a. Physical neglect, such as the lack of appropriate supervision or the failure to provide necessary food, shelter, or medical care.
  b. Educational neglect, such as failure to educate a child or attend to his/her special education needs.
  c. Emotional neglect, such as the inattention to a child's emotional needs or the exposure of a child to domestic violence.
  d. Excessive corporal punishment also is legally considered a form of neglect.

I suspect abuse but I don't have proof, should I report it?

New York State requires and school personnel to report child abuse. Usually, reasonable suspicion or reasonable cause to believe is enough for a person to report according to law. As a rule, when in doubt, report. Reporting is anonymous. Failure to report can result in criminal or civil liability.

What do I (mandated reporter) do before making a report?
  • Contact the Program Director. Make sure they are aware of your suspicion and that you are required by law to report your suspicion.
  • Document as much factual information as possible. Bruises, comments, disturbing or sexual writing or journaling, sexual themes in the play, how often the child comes hungry to school, etc.
  • Interview the child you suspect is being abused. Or have the director's designee conduct the interview. Ask open questions about what you've observed, but do not ask leading questions to the child.

Do ask open questions (i.e. So tell me, how did you get those bruises.).
Do not ask leading questions (i.e. So your Dad is abusing you, right?)
Let the child disclose to you what is happening. Be aware that they may not tell you the truth, and you should still disclose if you suspect they are hiding abuse.

How do I report abuse? Call 1- 800-342-3720

Accident Reporting Procedures

Any accident/injury serious or minor must be reported by completing the *YOUR ORGANIZATION's* Accident/Injury Form. The form should be completed within 24 hours of the injury.

REPORTING DEATH OR SERIOUS INJURY
The following procedures apply to adult leadership at the scene of a serious injury or fatality.
Most important, first care for the injured and prevent further injuries. Call 911 for help and
begin providing first aid. If the injury is life-threatening, call 911 first. Coaches/Adult volunteers are responsible for informing the Program Director or designee of a death or serious injury or illness as soon as possible. A serious injury or illness is defined as:
1. Any period of unconsciousness;
2. Any hospital inpatient admission; or
3. Any surgical intervention beyond suturing skin or setting simple fractures.
Leaders should be prepared to give specific facts regarding:
Who? Name and age of the subject, age, and name and complete address of parent(s) or next of kin.
When? Date, time of day
Where? Location and community
What? Nature of illness or accident
How? Illness/accident details, if known (e.g., swimming, boating, hiking)
Prompt and accurate reporting to the news media is most important. The local council has a
crisis communications plan, and the Scout executive will designate one spokesperson in order to avoid conflicting reports. Parents or next of kin will be informed by personal contact before any release is made to the public.

Evaluation of Coaches

It should be the goal every organization to provide the highest caliber volunteer coach for our youth. The expectation for a coach should be high in terms of performance and accountability. However, the organization shares the responsibility for bringing a coach to his or her maximum productivity by way of training and making resources available for advanced learning. Your organization should evaluate the coaching staff annually to determine their level of efficiency. In addition, every child and parent are encouraged to evaluate the coaches at the end of the season.

Complaint Procedure

Before filling out a complaint form it is important to remember the following:

The Name of Your Organization is a nonprofit organization operated by volunteers. Participating in *The Name of Your Organization* activities, as with any non-profit organization, is a privilege and not a right. **Anyone who cannot work cooperatively and is habitually disruptive – child or adult- will be asked to leave. In order to serve as an adult volunteer, you must be able to work cooperatively with others.**
Please keep to the issue and do not use this complaint form as a method to embarrass other coaches, volunteers, parents, or child participants. We want to solve problems in a constructive manner and not create new ones.

In addition, it is necessary for adult volunteers to:
- Be able to assess a potential problem and also view the problem from differing perspectives.
- Treat others with respect and consideration, whether or not the same courtesy is being extended to you.
- Recognize that families come from a variety of backgrounds and experiences and may view situations differently than you do, and with equal validity.
- Have the ability to objectively discuss problems in a positive manner without drawing in others or taking sides.

NOTE: *Using any kind of recording device without the prior consent of all parties is not acceptable. This equipment may be used only if all parties are informed and agree in advance.*

Steps in filing a complaint

Step One - Meet locally with the person(s) with whom you are having problems in a neutral and non-threatening environment. If you feel uncomfortable, ask a third person who is respected by both parties to serve as an objective mediator to keep the conversation on positive terms. ***The Name of Your Organization's* Staff will not discuss this issue until Step one (1) has been completed.**
Keep in mind that once a formal complaint has been filed, negative feelings may surface. It is not unusual for one or more people involved in the complaint to leave the program.
   Points to keep in mind while completing Step One
- Be civil *(No name calling or threats)*.
- List concerns on paper and go through each one.
- Listen openly and objectively to each other without interrupting.
- *The Name of Your Organization* is for everyone from all walks of life. Please set aside any differences you may have with other community members based on lifestyle, personalities, or previous experiences in other settings so positive cooperation for our youth can be modeled.
- Solutions are often made through compromises. In order for everyone to benefit from the experience, the outcome must be one where all parties agree.

If Step One fails to result in the resolution of the conflict, then the parties involved may proceed to Step Two.

Step Two - Fill out the attached complaint form. Be specific and offer positive solutions, (Note: removing people from the program is generally not a constructive solution). Try to be objective in stating the facts rather than making accusations.

Step Three - Send complaint copy to *The Name of Your Organization* and a copy to the person or persons who are listed on the complaint. The response must be in writing within seven days.

Step Four - *The Name of Your Organization* Board of Directors will review and assign an ad hoc committee if needed. *The Name of Your Organization* staff will review the complaint and responses(s) before approving action to be taken by Executive Board. Possible actions could be:
- Determining if there are grounds for any action.
- Meeting with all parties involved and working towards a positive solution if complaints are founded.

Step Five - If a solution cannot be reached, *The Name of Your Organization* Staff will request input from the Board of Directors who will make the final decision. Each party will be informed of the decision. If any of the parties do not honor the decision, **they will be asked to leave the program.**

Special thanks to the 4-H Club of Pleasant Hill, CA for providing this model.

Annual Calendar/Timeline

August
- Meet with school principal to discuss Saturday Program (Get key dates on school calendar)
- Begin to secure speakers for the Saturday Program
- Interview/screen prospective coaches
- Decide to secure the space needed for the Saturday Program
- Update website

September
- Distributing flyers about the program.
- Conduct registration
- Coaches Meeting/Training
- Secure insurance.
- Register and rate players
- Order uniforms
- Send out letters/invitations for "Coaches Who Cook"
- Update website

October

- Basketball Training Clinics
- Parents Orientation
- Draft for teams
- Release schedule for Parents Workshops
- Create schedule for guest speakers
- Coaches Training
- Update website

November
- Saturday Program begins
- Coaches Who Cook weekly promotions
- Racial and Cultural Harmony Day
- Weekly posting of "Player of the Week" on website
- Weekly Scope Standing Posted
- Order Trophies/Plagues

December
- Coaches Who Cook
- All-Stars Selected
- All-Star Game
- Awards Ceremony

Key Phone Numbers and Websites/Email Addresses

National Give Back for Kids Campaign	1-347-9743683	www.giveback4kids.org
Reporting Child Abuse in NYS	1-800-342-3720	www.ocfs.state.ny.us/main/cps/
Volunteer Screening	1-866.300.8524	www.backgroundchecks.com
CPR Training	1-877-REDCROSS	www.NYRedCross.org
K & K Insurance	866-554-4636	www.kandkinsurance.com
T-Shirts	718-708-4425	www.custom101prints.com
Trophies	718-824-4877	www.crowntrophy.com/stores-8
AAU Basketball	407-828-3197	www.aausports.org
42nd Precinct	718-402-3887	
Hosea James Givan II		hoseajg2@gmail.com
Coach Ted Gustus		www.theglobalmajoritycommunity.com
Positive Coaching Alliance		www.positivecoach.org
Junior NBA		http://jr.nba.com
Brooklyn Nets Academy		www.netsacademy.com
Junior Knicks		www.nba.com/knicks/junior/
Reviving Baseball in Inner Cities		www.mlb.com/rbi/
NFL Play Football		http://playfoot.nfl.com/
Major League Soccer New York City FC		www.nycfc.com/youth
US Youth Soccer Programs		www.usyouthsoccer.org
Junior Rangers Youth Hockey		www.nhl.com/rangers/community/youth-hockey
Ice Hockey in Harlem (NY Rangers)		www.nhl.com/rangers/community/ihih
WNBA/Jr NBA		https://jr.nba.com/hertimetoplay/
International Association of Approved Basketball Officials	717.713.8129	

Parent Rating Form

Week of:

Dear Parent,

As you know your son is a participant in the **2022 Saturday Spring League.** We have instituted the **S.C.O.P.E. System** (**S**chool and **C**hores **O**ptimizing **P**erformance **E**valuation). The system which is designed to assist parents and teachers toward instilling in children a sense of responsibility in the areas of academics and household chores. This concept supports the belief that "It takes a village to raise a child." This form is used to determine team standings, where the weight of the formula is placed on
academics, attendance, and chore responsibility, rather than winning or losing a basketball game. Thus, emphasizing *"the more important things in life."* Please complete your child's household chore performance by circling the number (1 being the lowest, 5 being the highest) that most accurately reflects this week's evaluation in the appropriate categories.
We are also asking you to sign at the bottom of the page. Thanks for allowing us to help!

Name of Player _____

Team _____

Attitude/Behavior	1 2 3 4 5	
Cleaned Room	1 2 3 4 5	
_____	1 2 3 4 5	
(Other Chore)		

_____

Parent Signature

HJG2-2021

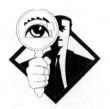

Name of Student _____   **Coach** _____

Team _____

Teacher Rating for Week of:

Teacher/Dean,
This student is a participant in the Saturday Spring League. We have instituted the **SCOPE** (**S**chool and **C**hores **O**ptimizing **P**erformance **E**valuation) **System.** It is designed to improve academic performance. Please help us monitor this student's classroom performance by circling the number (1 being the lowest, 5 being the highest) that most accurately reflects this week's evaluation in the appropriate categories. We are also asking each teacher to initial next to your subject. Thanks for your help!J

Attended Class	1 2 3 4 5
Had Work Materials	1 2 3 4 5
Paid Attention	1 2 3 4 5
Homework	1 2 3 4 5
Attitude	1 2 3 4 5

**For Office Use Only
Total Points _____**

HJG2-2021

VOLUNTEER COACH APPLICATION FORM

1. Name _____

1a). E-mail address _____

2. Address _____

3. Phone (Home) _____   (Work) _____

3a) Best time to be reached _____

4. Do you have coaching experience?   Yes_____   No_____

5. If so, please list the organization(s):_____

6. Please give the names and numbers of two references:

    a) Name _____ b) Phone _____

    b) Name _____ b) Phone _____

7. Will you be available every Saturday?   Yes _____ No _____

8. Do you have a son or daughter in the program?   Yes _____ No _____

8a) Name of child(ren) _____

9. What additional activities would you like to volunteer for?
o Security   o Score keeper
o Timekeeper   o Referee
o Fundraising   o Street crossing
o Concessions stand   o Assist with homework/tutor
o Life Skills presenter   o Administrative

10. How did you find out about the program? _____

11. Have you ever been convicted of a felony? If so, what crime? _____

12. Are you open to having a background check? Yes___ No___ Have you been fingerprinted? Yes___ No___

12. Are you willing to participate in a mandatory 6 hour volunteer training program? Yes___ No___

Signature _____   Date _____

VOLUNTEER FORM

1. Name _____

1a). E-mail address _____

2. Address _____ Apt/house # . _____

3. Phone (Home) _____ (Work) _____

3a) Best time to be reached _____

4. Do you have volunteer experience?   Yes_____   No_____

5. If so, please list the organization(s):

 a) _____
 b) _____

6. Please give the names and numbers of two references :

 a) Name _____ b) Phone _____
 b) Name _____ b) Phone _____

7. Will you be available every Saturday?   Yes _____ No _____

8. Do you have a son or daughter in the program?   Yes _____ No _____

8a) Name of child(ren) _____

9. What activity would you like to volunteer for?

o Security   o Score keeper   o Assist with homework
o Time keeper   o Referee   o Tutor
o Fundraising   o Street crossing   o Mentor
o Concession stand   o Dance instruction   o Computer Trainer/Mentor
o Life Skills presenter   o Administrative   o Other _____

10. How did you find out about the program? _____

11. Have you ever been convicted of a felony? If so, what crime? _____

12. Are you willing to participate in a mandatory 2 hour volunteer training program? Yes___ No___

Signature _____   Date _____

Registration and Waiver Form

Name of participant _____ ☐ Male ☐ Female

Address: _____ Home Phone:_____

_____ Date of Birth:_____ Age: _____

Name of Parent or Guardian: _____ Email:_____

Parent/Guardian's work phone;_____ Cell Phone: _____

In case of emergency, notify: _____ Emergency #: _____

Name of school:_____ Class:_____
Grade:_____

Height: _____ Weight:_____ Ethnicity: (optional) _____ T-shirt size: _____

Does your child take any medication or have any allergies?: _____

Please describe any chronic or recurring illnesses that your child has:_____

Does your child have any conditions that require activity to be restricted?:_____

Insurance carrier:_____ I.D.#/Medicaid #: _____

Parent Agreements

1. I hereby certify that I am parent or legal guardian of _____ (child's name)("Participant") and I am authorized to execute this registration and waiver on his/her behalf.

2. I hereby certify that the participant is in normal health and is capable of participating safely in the Saturday Spring League.

3. I hereby authorize Spring League Coordinators to act in my behalf in accordance with their best judgment in case of an emergency and to obtain necessary medical treatment for my child with the understanding that the family will be notified as soon as possible.

4. I, on my own behalf and behalf of Participant, hereby and forever release and discharge The Name of Your Sports League or Organization, another important sponsor, Department of Education, P.S. 000, of and the staff or volunteers of each and every one of the aforesaid entities against any and all causes of action, claims, suits, controversies, agreements, promises, judgments, demands or claims whatsoever, that I or my spouse, heirs, executors, administrators, successors or assigns have or hereafter, at any time, shall or may have arisen due to negligence or otherwise.

5. In consideration of the goodwill, public service, and community aid provided by Saturday Spring League, which I support and from which I have received a benefit, I hereby grant permission of Saturday Spring League to use Participant's name, to take and publish photographs, videotapes or motion pictures of him/her which may include his/her voice, in any media for a legitimate purpose. I release all rights to such photographs, videotapes, motion pictures, and recordings. I acknowledge you are the sole owner of all rights arising out of their use for all purposes. I understand that I shall receive no compensation for their use from any source whatsoever.

6. I have read the Code of Behavior for participants and understand that if my child does not maintain these standards, he/she will forfeit his/her involvement with the program.

_____ _____
Signature of Parent/Guardian Date

(YOUR LOGO)

Each child will be expected to honor 4 commitments:

1. Get educated enough to establish a career or business.

2. When you're able to help others, GIVE BACK!

3. Be a good father (or mother) and be a good role model.

4. Maintain a healthy mind, body and spirit.

Our commitments to them:

1. Each child in our program will feel loved and respected.

2. Each child will have an organization they will always belong to.

3. Each child will learn important things they may not learn in school.

4. Each child will be taught about the importance of being a leader.

Saturday Spring League Schedule (Sample)

Nov. 11th

9:00am – 9:15am   Opening Prayer and Announcements

9:20am – 10:15am   Future Stars (Gymnasium)
Next Level (Cafeteria) – Guest Speaker Coach Robert Greene (Topic - Balancing Basketball, Books and God)

10:20am – 11:05am   Future Stars (Cafeteria) – Guest Speaker Coach Robert Greene (Topic - Balancing Basketball, Books and God)
Game 1 Next Level (Gymnasium)
Game 2 Next Level (Room 105 – Coach Time)
Bye Team (Room 106 – Coach Time)

11:10am – 11:55am   Future Stars Game 1 (Cafeteria East – Coach Time)
Future Stars Game 2 (Cafeteria West – Coach Time)
Next Level Losing Team (Room 105 – Coach Time)
Next Level Winning Team (Room 106 – Coach Time)

Nov. 18th

9:00am – 9:15am   Opening Prayer and Announcements

9:20am – 10:15am   Future Stars (Gymnasium)
Next Level (Cafeteria) – Guest Speaker Rachel Cheeks (Topic - Health & Wellness)

10:20am – 11:05am   Future Stars (Cafeteria) – Guest Speaker Rachel Cheeks (Topic - Health & Wellness)
Game 1 Next Level (Gymnasium)
Game 2 Next Level (Room 105 – Coach Time)
Bye Team (Room 106 – Coach Time)

11:10am – 11:55am   Future Stars Game 1 (Cafeteria East – Coach Time)
Future Stars Game 2 (Cafeteria West – Coach Time)
Next Level Losing Team (Room 105 – Coach Time)
Next Level Winning Team (Room 106 – Coach Time)

Dec. 2nd

9:00am – 9:15am   Opening Prayer and Announcements

9:20am – 10:15am   Future Stars All-Star Game (Gymnasium)
Next Level (Cafeteria) – Guest Speaker Bruce Bishop (Topic – Preparing for Success in Sports)

10:20am – 11:05am   Future Stars (Cafeteria) – Guest Speaker Bruce Bishop (Topic – Preparing for Success in Sports
Game 1 Next Level (Gymnasium)
Game 2 Next Level (Room 105 – Coach Time)
Bye Team (Room 106 – Coach Time)

11:10am – 11:55am   Future Stars Game 1 (Cafeteria East – Coach Time)
Future Stars Game 2 (Cafeteria West – Coach Time)
Next Level Losing Team (Room 105 – Coach Time)
Next Level Winning Team (Room 106 – Coach Time)

Parent Training Workshops

1. Families involvement with Government Systems
Objective - Workshop participants will learn about statistics from government systems and how they are impacting families. Participants will learn skills to prevent and avoid being a negative statistic and take ownership of parental responsibilities and their family's wellbeing.

2. Organizing Your Life Now and Planning for Your Family's Future.
Objective - Workshop participants will learn the necessary skills to organize their daily lives, how to set goals and reach them and how to plan for their families economic future. Participants will learn how to build internal systems within their household and set structure; provide healthy supervision and monitoring for their families outcomes.

3. Community Resources
Objective - Workshop participants will learn what community services are, how to find them and the importance of accessing them for their family's future.

4. Self Sufficiency Life Skills Information
Objective - Workshop participants will learn why education in various topics greatly affects their family's financial future (post-secondary education/trade training, career choices and employment benefits, basic budgeting, savings and retirement planning, family planning and the importance of becoming healthy and how to make lifestyle changes).

5. Parenting
Workshop participants will learn to take an active role in their parenting journey. Participants will build communication skills within the family.

6. Becoming Your Best Advocate
Objective - Workshop participants will learn how to handle the stress associated with advocating for benefits, services and flaws in government systems that affect families' lives (public entitlement programs, child support, housing, medical coverage, domestic violence, etc.).

7. Maintaining a Healthy Mind and Body is Essential in Good Parenting
Objective – Workshop participants will be provided helpful information in regard to maintaining a healthy, mind, body and spirit.

8. Living in a Post Coronavirus World
Objective – Workshop participants will better understand the ways in that the Coronavirus has changed society.

Partial Listing of Past Workshop Facilitators:
Person A
Person B
Person C
Person D
Person E

Game Day Organization Sheet

Date_____

☐ Front Door Security Name_____
　　　　　　　　　　　　　　　　　Name_____
　　　　　　　　　　　　　　　　　Name_____

☐ 3rd Floor Security　Name_____

☐ Life Skills Speakers Name_____
　　　　Name_____

☐ Scorekeeper Game 1　　Name_____
☐ Timekeeper Game 1　　　　Name_____
☐ Official　　　　　　　　　　Name_____
☐ Official　　　　　　　　　　Name_____

☐ Scorekeeper Game 2　　Name_____
☐ Timekeeper Game 2　　　　Name_____
☐ Official　　　　　　　　　　Name_____
☐ Official　　　　　　　　　　Name_____

☐ Scorekeeper Game 3　　Name_____
☐ Timekeeper Game 3　　　　Name_____
☐ Official　　　　　　　　　　Name_____
☐ Official　　　　　　　　　　Name_____

☐ Scorekeeper Game 4　　Name_____
☐ Timekeeper Game 4　　　　Name_____
☐ Official　　　　　　　　　　Name_____
☐ Official　　　　　　　　　　Name_____

Overall Stat Sheet

Game Info   **Date_____**

Future Stars Division

Winner Score Team_____	Amount U	Loser Score Team_____	Amount U
Top Scorer Name _____		Top Scorer Name _____	
Assist Leader Name _____		Assist Leader Name _____	
Blocked Shots Leader Name _____		Blocked Shots Leader Name _____	
Top Rebounder Name _____		Top Rebounder Name _____	
Steals Leader Name _____		Steals Leader Name _____	

Winner Score Team_____	Amount U	Loser Score Team_____	Amount U
Top Scorer Name _____		Top Scorer Name _____	
Assist Leader Name _____		Assist Leader Name _____	
Blocked Shots Leader Name _____		Blocked Shots Leader Name _____	
Top Rebounder Name _____		Top Rebounder Name _____	
Steals Leader Name _____		Steals Leader Name _____	

Overall Stat Sheet #2

Game Info   **Date_____**

Next Level Division

Winner Score Team_____	Amount Ʊ	Loser Score Team_____	Amount Ʊ
Top Scorer Name _____		Top Scorer Name _____	
Assist Leader Name _____		Assist Leader Name _____	
Blocked Shots Leader Name _____		Blocked Shots Leader Name _____	
Top Rebounder Name _____		Top Rebounder Name _____	
Steals Leader Name _____		Steals Leader Name _____	

Winner Score Team_____	Amount Ʊ	Loser Score Team_____	Amount Ʊ
Top Scorer Name _____		Top Scorer Name _____	
Assist Leader Name _____		Assist Leader Name _____	
Blocked Shots Leader Name _____		Blocked Shots Leader Name _____	
Top Rebounder Name _____		Top Rebounder Name _____	
Steals Leader Name _____		Steals Leader Name _____	

Individual Statistics

Game Stats   Date_____ Team _____

Team_____ vs. Team_____

#	Name	Rebounds	Assists	Steals	Blocked Shots

PLAYER SKILL EVALUATION

Evaluation Scale: 5 = Excellent, 4 = Above Average, 3 = Average, 2 = Below Average, 1 = Unskilled

INDIVIDUAL FUNDAMENTAL SKILLS	CIRCLE RATING					COMMENTS
SHOOTING	5	4	3	2	1	
ONE-ON-ONE SKILLS	5	4	3	2	1	
PASSING/BALL HANDLING (Dribbling)	5	4	3	2	1	
OFFENSIVE & DEFENSIVE MOVEMENT WITHOUT THE BALL (Screening, cutting, etc.)	5	4	3	2	1	
REBOUNDING	5	4	3	2	1	
DEFENSE: BALL & OFF THE BALL	5	4	3	2	1	
OTHER EVALUATION AREAS:						
COACHABLITY: (Listening to and doing what coach says)	5	4	3	2	1	
WORK ETHIC	5	4	3	2	1	
HUSTLE/AGGRESSIVENESS	5	4	3	2	1	
TEAM PLAYER	5	4	3	2	1	
MAINTENANCE PROGRAM (1) BEGINNERS (2) INTERMEDIATE (3) ADVANCED						
SHOOTING		1		2	3	
BALL HANDLING		1		2	3	
REBOUNDING		1		2	3	
FOOTWORK/CONDITIONING		1		2	3	
ADDITIONAL COMMENTS:						

Basketball Score Sheet

Team _____

Coach _____

Date _____

1 2 3 4 5 6 7 8 9 10 11 12 13 14 15 16 17 18 19 20 21 22 23 24 25 26 27 28 29 30 31 32 33 34 35 36 37 38 39 40 41 42 43 44 45 46 47 48 49 50 51 52 53 54 55

56 57 58 59 60 61 62 63 64 65 66 67 68 69 70 71 72 73 74 75 76 77 78 79 80 81 82 83 84 85 86 87 88 89 90 91 92 93 94 95 96 97 98 99 100 101 102 103 104

105 106 107 108 109 110 111 112 113 114 115 116 117 118 119 120

TIME-OUTS: (FULL) ❶ ❷ ❸ (20 SEC.) ❶ ❷ (OVERTIME) ❶ ❷   **WARNING:** ❶   **TEAM FOULS:** 1 2 3 4 5 6 7 8 9 10

PLAYER	NO.	FOULS	1ST QUARTER	2ND QUARTER	3RD QUARTER	4TH QUARTER	TOTAL
		1 2 3 4 5					
		1 2 3 4 5					
		1 2 3 4 5					
		1 2 3 4 5					
		1 2 3 4 5					
		1 2 3 4 5					
		1 2 3 4 5					
		1 2 3 4 5					
		1 2 3 4 5					
		1 2 3 4 5					
		1 2 3 4 5					
		1 2 3 4 5					
		1 2 3 4 5					
		1 2 3 4 5					
		1 2 3 4 5					

HJG2021©

Coach Evaluation

Coach: _____ (1 form per coach)

Division: _____

Coach Evaluation Questionnaire--For PLAYERS

The National Give Back for Kids Campaign, Inc. supports the Positive Coaching Alliance ideals. Please help us evaluate how well we did this season by telling us about your coaches. We want our coaches to be "Double-Goal Coaches" who strive to win and to help players learn lessons that will help them be successful in life.

A Positive Coach:
• **Honors the Game** by showing respect for the rules, opponents, officials, teammates and oneself.
• **Redefines "Winner"** in terms of Mastery as well as the scoreboard by emphasizing effort, learning and improvement, and rebounding from mistakes rather than fearing them.
• **Fills "Emotional Tanks"** via positive encouragement so players can play their best.

My coach…	Strongly Disagree						Strongly Agree

Honoring the Game

1) Obeyed the rules	1	2	3	4	5	6	7
2) Showed respect for officials	1	2	3	4	5	6	7
3) Treated all players with respect	1	2	3	4	5	6	7
4) Treated opponents with respect	1	2	3	4	5	6	7

Redefined "Winner"

5) Rewarded effort, not just results	1	2	3	4	5	6	7
6) Helped players learn and improve in the sport	1	2	3	4	5	6	7
7) Helped players bounce back from mistakes	1	2	3	4	5	6	7

Filling Emotional Tanks

8) Had a nurturing and loving demeanor	1	2	3	4	5	6	7
9) Used positive reinforcement	1	2	3	4	5	6	7
10) Encouraged players to do their best	1	2	3	4	5	6	7
11) Made the sport fun for me	1	2	3	4	5	6	7
12) Listened to players	1	2	3	4	5	6	7

13) Would you like to play for this coach again?   Yes   No

Feel free to use the back for comments. (*Special thanks to the Foster City Little League (Foster City, California*

Coach Evaluation

Coach: _____ (1 form per coach)

Division: _____

Coach Evaluation Questionnaire--For PARENTS

The National Give Back for Kids Campaign, Inc. supports the Positive Coaching Alliance ideals. Please help us evaluate how well we did this season by telling us about your coaches. We want our coaches to be "Double-Goal Coaches" who strive to win and to help players learn lessons that will help them be successful in life.

A Positive Coach:
• **Honors the Game** by showing respect for the rules, opponents, officials, teammates and oneself.
• **Redefines "Winner"** in terms of Mastery as well as the scoreboard by emphasizing effort, learning and improvement, and rebounding from mistakes rather than fearing them.
• **Fills "Emotional Tanks"** via positive encouragement so players can play their best.

My child's coach…	Strongly Disagree						Strongly Agree

Honoring the Game

1) Obeyed the rules	1	2	3	4	5	6	7
2) Showed respect for officials	1	2	3	4	5	6	7
3) Treated all players with respect	1	2	3	4	5	6	7
4) Treated opponents with respect	1	2	3	4	5	6	7

Redefined "Winner"

5) Rewarded effort, not just results	1	2	3	4	5	6	7
6) Helped players learn and improve in the sport	1	2	3	4	5	6	7
7) Helped players bounce back from mistakes	1	2	3	4	5	6	7

Filling Emotional Tanks

8) Had a nurturing and loving demeanor	1	2	3	4	5	6	7
9) Used positive reinforcement	1	2	3	4	5	6	7
10) Encouraged players to do their best	1	2	3	4	5	6	7
11) Made the sport fun for me	1	2	3	4	5	6	7
12) Listened to players	1	2	3	4	5	6	7

13) Would you like to play for this coach again?   Yes   No

Feel free to use the back for comments. (*Special thanks to the Foster City Little League (Foster City, California)*

Volunteer Protection Act

In 1997, President Clinton signed into law the Volunteer Protection Act of 1997 that, generally speaking, provides immunity from tort claims that might be filed against the volunteers of nonprofit organizations. When an individual performs volunteer services for a non-profit he exposes himself to the risk of having a claim filed against him by someone who believes he has been hurt by the volunteer. The Volunteer Protection Act provides immunity from lawsuits filed against a nonprofit's volunteer where the claim is that he carelessly injured another in the course of helping the nonprofit.

Public Law 105-19; the Volunteer Protection Act of 1997 as signed into law by President Clinton on June 18, 1997
C. Volunteer Protection Act of 1997:

The **Volunteer** Protection Act of 1997 (42 U.S.C. 14501, et. seq.) is a federal law which preempts **state** law, except where the **state** law provides additional protection from **liability** relating to **volunteers** or to any category of **volunteers** in the performance of services for a nonprofit organization or governmental entity. Generally, the Act provides that no volunteer of a nonprofit organization or governmental entity shall be liable for harm caused by an act or omission of the volunteer on behalf of the organization or entity if:
1) The volunteer was acting within the scope of his or her responsibilities at the time of the act or omission.
2) If appropriate or required, the volunteer was properly licensed, certified, or authorized in the state in which the harm occurred, where the activities were or practice was undertaken within the scope of the volunteer's responsibilities.
3) The harm was not the result of willful or criminal misconduct, gross negligence, reckless misconduct, or a conscious flagrant indifference to the rights or safety of the individual harmed by the volunteer; and,
4) The harm was not caused by the volunteer's operation of a motor vehicle, vessel, aircraft or other vehicle for which the state requires the operator or the owner of the vehicle, craft or vessel to a) possess an operator's license or b) maintain insurance. Generally, punitive damages may not be awarded against a volunteer in an action brought for harm based on the action of a volunteer acting within the scope of the volunteer's responsibilities to a nonprofit organization or governmental entity unless the claimant establishes by clear and convincing evidence that the harm was proximately caused by an action of such volunteer which constitutes willful or criminal misconduct, or a conscious, flagrant indifference to the rights or safety of the individual harmed. The limitations on liability do not apply to any misconduct that:
1) constitutes a crime of violence (as defined in Section 16 of Title 18. United States ~) or act of international terrorism (as that term is defined in Section 2331 of Title ~), for which the defendant has been convicted in any court;
2) constitutes a hate crime (as that term is used in the Hate Crime Statistics Act (~ U.S.C. 534);
3) involves a sexual offense, as defined by applicable state law, for which the person has been convicted in any court;
4) involves misconduct for which the defendant has been found to have violated a federal or state civil rights law; or,
5) where the person was under the influence (as determined under applicable state law) of intoxicating alcohol or any drug at the time of the misconduct.

(YOUR LOGO)

Complaint Form

Name:

Home Address:

Telephone:

E-mail:

Description of Complaint (please be as specific as possible in describing the event(s), date(s), person(s) involved, etc.):

Proposed remedy:

Signature	Date

Use of this form is voluntary. Return this signed and dated.

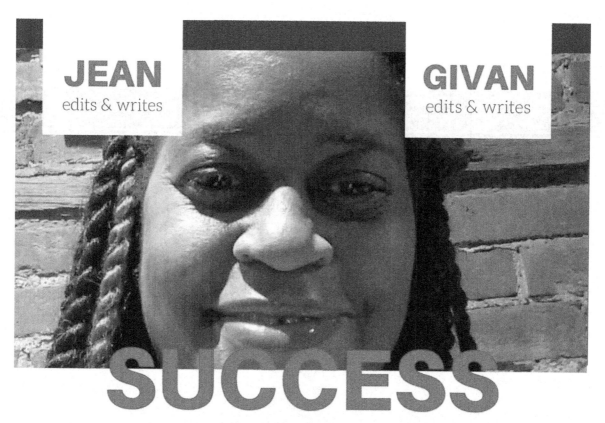

JEAN
edits & writes

GIVAN
edits & writes

SUCCESS

FOR YOUR WRITING PROJECT
Just a Phone Call or Email Away

Got You Covered

Backed with a BA degree in English from Syracuse University and decades of experierience

Innovative Ideas

Will help you in writing by delivering good ideas and strategies. It is easy to succeed with Jean's help

Key to Success

Taking action with someone who can help you manage your writing all the way to the top

Clients Choose Jean!

Easy but professional flow from start to finish, from an idea to published book with ease. Effort necessary but not complicated.

Call Jean (516) 688-5497 or Send an Email:
jean@personalizedbyjean.com

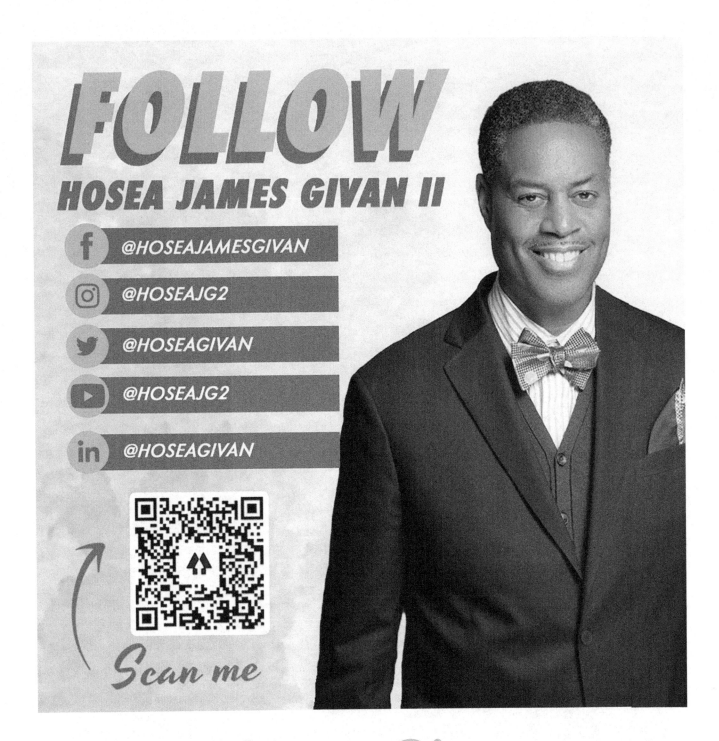

www.HoseaGivan.com

Email: info@hoseagivan.com

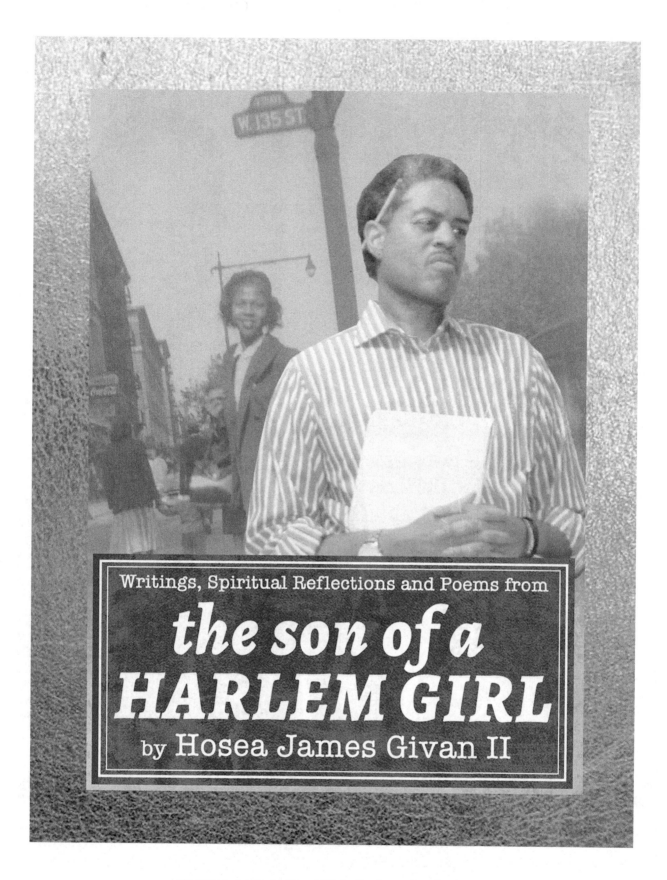

Writings, Spiritual Reflections and Poems from

the son of a
HARLEM GIRL

by Hosea James Givan II

COMING FALL 2021

Made in the USA
Middletown, DE
08 May 2021